I Foug̶̶ ̶t̶h̶e̶ ̶L̶a̶w̶ ̶(̶A̶n̶d̶ the Law Won)

A Collection of Reader-Submitted Medical Stories

LEO EDITION

Kerry Hamm

Disclaimer:

Names, locations, and portions of the
details included in this book have been altered
to protect the privacy of those involved.

Warning:

This edition features light profanity that may be offensive to some readers. The profanity has been used sparingly and in each instance the usage was included in the submission. I have chosen to leave some of these words in to emphasize portions of the stories.

By now, I am sure you are all too familiar with my *Real Stories from a Small-Town ER* series, which were collections of stories told to you from my time as a registration clerk in Ohio. If you are new here, don't fret! You don't have to worry about a 'certain order' for *any* of my books, including this one!

I have since moved on from the hospital scene, but that hasn't stopped readers from submitting stories of their own experiences from the medical field. Over time, I have received hundreds of stories-some funny, some sad, some downright scary or grotesque-and have worked with my readers to bring these stories to you in a follow up to my last *Real Stories* volume.

If I've learned anything from writing my series and compiling this book, it's that none of us are alone. We're all proof that we've seen some seriously messed up things out there, right? We have seen the good. We've seen the bad. We've seen the downright vile and disgusting. And then, we've seen the humor in these situations and we've been fortunate enough to share them with one another. There is a certain peace in knowing that as no matter how crazy we feel, we have formed solidarity amongst ourselves, knowing that for every bad day you've had, others have had them too. We have worked through the challenges of getting up and facing another drug seeker, another child abuse case, another young death, and another 'how the heck did that even happen?' moment together. You guys are not alone, and this book reaffirms that.

Several of the stories have been edited to bring you clear-cut and clean versions of tales submitted by loyal readers. I have done my very best to edit out hospital and town names, and in some cases my submitters wished to withhold their initials and other details from publication or requested that I edit stories for grammar/spelling. Some stories have been edited for length. I do my very best to preserve a reader's humor and emotions, as well as capture the reader's personality when I edit these submissions.

Though some of the stories in this collection are horrifying, I am glad none of us are alone in what we've witnessed or experienced.

<u>Cheat Sheet</u>

Some readers have been confused about terms used in this series. Here's a quick list to help you out!

LEO: Law Enforcement Officer

ETOH: shorthand for Ethyl Alcohol or Ethanol; commonly used to describe intoxicated individuals

Bus/Rig/Truck: Ambulance

M.D.: Medical Doctor

R.N.: Registered Nurse

MVA: Motor Vehicle Accident

EMS: Emergency Medical Services

EMT: Emergency Medical Technician

PD/FD: Police Department/Fire Department

D.A.: District Attorney

BOLO: Be on (the) Lookout

DCFS/CPS: Department of Children and Family Services/Child Protective Services

SNF: Skilled Nursing Facility. This can be a nursing home or facilities for patients in need of supervised care

AMA: Against Medical Advice

Let's Not Have It Your Way

On my first day back following a surgical procedure, I'm positively certain a higher power decided to throw at me every last bit of drama I had missed during the six weeks I had spent on the couch.

I was called to respond to a traffic stop before I had even cranked up the engine. That stop resulted in deploying a taser after our (inebriated) driver refused to comply with simple instructions. This occurred in the first 20 minutes of my shift, and I (stupidly) volunteered to escort the subject to the ER for a med-clearance prior to jail transport.

During the three-hour stretch the subject and I were in the emergency room, I participated in restraining the subject for inappropriate and violent behavior. The events leading up to restraint were as follows: the subject spit continually on nursing staff and kicked over a supply tray; the subject agreed to supply a urine sample and was urinating into a handheld plastic urinal, when he decided to 'whip it out' and piss down the front of my pants; the subject attempted to bolt as I was in the process of wiping piss from my pants; when the subject ran, he decided to fight with the hospital's security team for good measure—he was tased by the hospital security team when he picked up a syringe from a nearby cart and attempted to stab another ER patient. Once the subject was restrained, I admittedly felt immense relief, but I knew I would still have to transport the asshole and put up with him while he was in our facility's care. I hoped the subject's behavior would calm as he came down from the drugs and alcohol in his system.

As I was transporting the subject to jail, a garbage truck T-boned my vehicle. The driver had been distracted. Luckily, my subject waived his right to return to the ER, and I was uninjured. A fellow officer reported the incident and the subject was transported to jail. I was transferred to a 'spare' patrol unit. I'm pretty sure this car sat widely unused for several reasons, those of them being: a strong vibration in the steering wheel when the vehicle idled or I applied the brakes; brakes squealing so loudly that they could be heard over the sounds of illegal fireworks (literally, I responded to this call shortly after noon); and a heavy thumping sound/feeling from the tires when I would attempt to accelerate beyond 35 MPH. I will add that I spilled coffee on my recently-changed slacks. My day was not going well.

Near shift change, which I was highly anticipating, I was the lucky winner of "37, you're the only officer in the vicinity" of an altercation at a local fast food establishment. Several callers had reported to our 911 operator that two female employees were involved in a physical altercation and "it [was] bad." As with your stories of what a professional deems 'bad' versus what civilians deem 'bad,' I was left to believe the severity of the altercation had been slightly exaggerated.

Nope!

Upon entering the lobby of the restaurant, I immediately took note of spilled tea and soft drinks that had spread from the beverage station and all the way to the door. Packets of salt, ketchup, and barbeque sauce were scattered and largely busted and smeared in the sticky tea/soda mess. There was food on the floor and counter. A register was barely hanging on to the countertop, and its contents had been strewn in front of the ordering area and behind the register. Several patrons (all of whom had retreated to one side of the lobby) approached me with cell phones to show me videos. Some were still recording and panned over and proceeded with commentary for their videos.

The sounds from the kitchen were unbelievable. I could clearly make out several female voices hollering at one another. I could also hear a few male voices shouting. In addition to the screams, I heard pots and pans crashing down, and as I made my way to the kitchen, I was nearly crushed under a metal tower that had been pushed over. I proceeded around the tower to find a disgruntled woman who possessed no respect or fear of law enforcement. As I was attempting to subdue her, she hit, kicked, and even bit me. At this point, I was bleeding, and she was calling for help.

When patrons viewed this behavior, two stepped in and attempted to assist me. We moved the female employee to the ground and I cuffed her. No sooner than I felt the second cuff click, another assailant assaulted me. I think I took a spatula to the head. I requested one of the assisting patrons place a call to 911 and request all available officers to the establishment, with the current responding officer's safety in question. While the patron was placing this call, I was forced to deploy pepper spray on the spatula-wielder and another female employee.

Officers arrived within 15-minutes of the patron's 911 call, and by this time, I had wrestled subjects to the ground in both the kitchen and the lobby. I was soaked in soft drinks and had French fries and hamburger buns stuck to my uniform. My head was sore from the spatula-hit, and my hand was bleeding from where I had been bitten. Pepper spray had somehow transferred from a subject's skin to my own, and I managed to rub some of the residue in my own eyes, rendering myself partially-blind during this battle.

We determined the altercation began when a male entered the establishment and placed an order. Female A warmly greeted this man as her boyfriend. Female B heard the man's voice and approached the register. She, too, acknowledged the male as her boyfriend. What started as a verbal spew between the women escalated quickly into a full-out brawl. As other employees attempted to break up the fight, they too became involved in the violence.

What I found most offensive about this scene was not that I was assaulted or bitten (which required another ER visit that cut into what was supposed to be my time to relax after a day of work)—some people don't trust law enforcement and they have their reasons; I am mostly understanding of this and try to respectfully communicate my good intentions, so long as there is no violence involved. So that, I could understand. What I could not understand is how one of the female employees screamed to high heaven and refused arrest (and was ultimately tasered), and ONLY THEN did she notify officers that her CHILDREN were seated at a booth in the corner of the lobby and had witnessed the entire scene unfold.

Child Services took temporary custody of the employee's children, until they were released to another family member.

This happened a few years ago, but every now and then I see clips from this altercation floating around on social media.

--A.B.

Location withheld at request

*Author's Note: The title of this submission should not be accepted as a link to where the story took place. The title was purely selected for entertainment value.

<u>Hot Dogs</u>

Some time back, a peculiar crime plagued our rural community. On day one, we didn't think much of this, except, 'Well, that was weird.'

During that call, we assisted an elderly woman in filing a report because her (mostly outside) dog had allegedly been approached by an individual and its fur had been smothered in mayonnaise. The dog was uninjured, but every inch of its fur had been coated in mayo, and I couldn't imagine having the task of bathing the dog.

Again, we just found that to be 'weird.' Honestly, we thought this was a prank that would go unsolved. Some of us figured one of the elderly woman's neighbors did this to the dog, as a non-harmful way to coax the woman in bringing the dog in at night. We had no confirmed sighting of an individual performing this strange crime, so we basically didn't think too much more of it.

Two days later, we were called out to another residence. A man stated he had let his dogs outside in broad daylight so he could finish painting the basement. He said he heard his dogs bark a few times, but he thought nothing of it because they barked frequently at stray cats and squirrels. When the man went to let the dogs inside, he thought they had been injured or had injured another animal. Both dogs were found smothered in ketchup. This complainant was fuming, and I couldn't say that I blamed him.

Our officers started to question neighbors and attempt to pinpoint local hooligans who were regularly on our radar. With no evidence and no admissions of guilt, we couldn't do anything to help these canine owners. All we could do was file reports after-the-fact.

Over the course of a week, we responded to approximately a dozen more calls. We deemed the criminal the 'Canine Condiment Coverer' (I didn't say it was a great name, just what we came up with), as he/she had coated each of the dogs in condiments. I think we saw dogs covered in mayonnaise, ketchup, mustard, BBQ sauce, ranch dressing, and horseradish. Except for the dog who was covered in horseradish (who consumed the condiment from his fur and ended up at the vet for a bad bout of diarrhea), none of the animals were injured.

The last report of the Canine Condiment Coverer was taken from our humane shelter. Three dogs had been covered in mayonnaise. In addition, the dogs had been released from their outdoor pens and were found running through a nearby field when volunteers arrived for their shifts the next morning.

We received security camera footage from the humane shelter, but we could not get a lead on the criminal because he/she wore all-black attire, wore a mask and gloves, and once he/she noticed the cameras, he/she turned away from them and never faced them again.

Following our release of the footage to local news outlets, we didn't have another incident. I think about this often and would just be satisfied in knowing why someone would do this.

--J.P.

Indiana

<u>Help!</u>

Our rural station received a 911 call from a male at approximately 6 PM. He stated he had sustained an injury and needed 'all departments' to assist. The man stated he was on a boat, floating down the river, and he couldn't pinpoint his exact location. He stated his injury prevented him from starting the boat's motor or bringing himself back to shore. None of this was deemed unusual to our department. We routinely get calls from drunks or idiots who get lost on the river. We started charging a 'recovery fee' to cut down on having to waste our time bringing these imbeciles back.

An operator stayed on the line with the man and attempted to narrow his location. During the time, the man refused to discuss his injury, but he said he needed medical transport. There were times that he wept uncontrollably and the operator could not understand him.

After roughly an hour and a half, our officers tracked down the man to an obscure location. He had somehow ended up in what we call a 'dead zone' of the river, a location that has one entrance/exit, is usually difficult to navigate, and is stagnant. These areas are generally covered in algae/scum, and I can't say I've ever caught anything decent in a dead zone, but I've seen more than my fair share of gators and the kind of snakes you don't even want to look at. We call it a dead zone for more than one reason.

Our guys found the caller passed out on the floor of his boat. It was an odd sight. The man's pants were pulled down and he had his hands clamped to his genitals. There was blood…and beer cans… all over.

Upon closer examination, we saw the man's scrotum had been…torn would be the delicate way to explain this, but that wouldn't be accurate. It looked like someone had taken one of those bean bag sacks from cornhole and tried to cut it open with a serrated knife. A few of us guys had to get off his boat and some of the guys were puking off the side of our boats. I, for one, can say I've never seen anything like this before, and I never want to again. As a man, I'm scarred by this, and I'm not joking.

We met paramedics at a private dock about five miles away and the man was transported to the hospital, where he received an emergency blood transfusion after losing so much of his own blood.

From what we could gather about this incident, the man had somehow managed to hook himself in the testicles. He attempted to remove the hook from his jeans and scrotum, but couldn't, so he then attempted to pull down his pants and when he felt his skin tearing, he panicked. In a drunken state, he toppled over his fishing pole and basically ripped the hook from his skin.

Our city council (made up of many of the men who responded to this call) waived the fees we normally charge for a water-call, based on an agreement that the man already suffered enough.

I'm telling you, you really don't appreciate what you have until you see someone else going without. I'll remember this call for the rest of my life.

--O.T.

Alabama

I'm So Excited

As an officer formerly employed in the Las Vegas area, I can assure you I am no stranger to responding to calls from Gentleman's Clubs. When I moved to the Midwest, I thought my days of responding to these locations were long gone, but this proved me wrong.

I arrived on scene to a panicked dancer explaining to me that she, at the request of a young male's friends, had escorted a subject to the VIP corner of the club. The two entered a private room and the dancer began her one-on-one show for the young man. She stated he attempted to touch her, but she explained the experience was hands-off.

The dancer then explained that she had moved to perform a lap dance for her customer. When she placed her breasts near his face, the subject apparently gripped one of her breasts, and in return she slapped him. The 18 or 19-year-old slumped in the chair, and was called in as 'unresponsive.'

While I was waiting for medics to arrive, I slapped at the teen's cheeks a bit, until he came to. He sprang to life immediately and demanded that the dancers and his friends (who'd gathered to watch the panic) leave the area.

Once I was alone with the man, he explained his religious upbringing and stated this was the first time he had seen breasts in 'real life,' as opposed to viewing pornography. The teen stated he had felt his face grow hot and his heart thump away, before he tried to 'grab something' for leverage.

This young man pleaded with me not to tell the dancers or his friends what happened. It was difficult to watch because he was almost crying, begging me to lie.

I decided to do the young man a solid by pulling a medic aside and announcing to the crowd that the young man had blood sugar issues and simply needed to eat supper.

--T.E.

Iowa

If I pull you over and ask what that white powder is in that plastic baggy on your passenger seat and you answer, "Not drugs," I'm going to automatically assume you have a bag of drugs next to you.

Felony charges convicted in court: illegal possession of an unlicensed firearm by a felon, possession of cocaine in an amount >2 grams, intent to deliver, illegal operation of a vehicle while suspended, and no insurance. Charges dismissed: speeding (10-14 MPH over posted limit).

--N.Z.

Michigan

<u>Nothing to See Here, Folks</u>

Police officers put their lives on the line daily. These brave men and women encounter violent criminals on a regular basis and ask for nothing more than safety for themselves and others in return. Sometimes, though…Well, mistakes are made. Here are few accounts from officers who have responded to calls that required no intervention from law enforcement.

■■■■■■■■■■■■■■■■■■■■■■■■■■■■■■■■■■■■■■

Our station was bombarded with calls from bystanders at our local mall. We understood two males had placed an adult male and an adult female under citizen's arrest for the allegations of throwing an infant. You read that right… Callers stated they witnessed the male subject throw an infant through the air, and the female subject then threw the baby into the car. Whew, this was going to be something.

When I arrived, the subjects were obviously upset and so were all the witnesses. It took a few minutes to calm the lynch mob forming around the subjects' vehicle. These people were ready to perform street justice, and the scene was tense.

"We have reports that you threw a child," I said to the male subject.

"I told these damn people that it was a doll. It-was-a-DOLL!"

The female subject then lifted a life-like baby doll from the back seat and showed me. I had never seen a doll so life-like. Its hair looked real. It was weighted to feel like a real baby. Its skin was made of a soft silicone substance. Its facial features were molded perfectly. If I had seen still shots of this doll, I would have assumed it was a living, breathing newborn.

From the backseat, a *real* newborn cried. Mom lifted the child and attempted to calm the baby.

Our witnesses weren't taking this explanation lightly. We called in a medic team to perform a quick examination of the real baby. Somewhere along this timeline, someone had contacted Children and Family Services. An agent responded to the parking lot and demanded the child be transported to the emergency room for a documented wellness check. The parents were irate at this point, and I have to say that I couldn't blame them one bit because I believed their story, but the two agreed to a wellness check.

While the parents were at the hospital, we pulled security footage from the mall parking lot and indeed witnessed the mother placing the real baby inside the car. The father tossed the life-like doll through the air by its leg, and the mother then carelessly tossed the toy in the backseat. Within seconds of these actions, witnesses had surrounded the couple and prevented the couple from leaving.

After speaking to all parties, we all agreed this was a simple misunderstanding. The parents were wonderful through this and stated they did not wish to press charges on anyone because they would have done the same thing if they had been on the other side of the fence. Still, I can't help but to feel sorry for all the drama and stress the couple endured during the investigation.

--C.P.

Illinois

■■■

I was first on-scene to reports of a suicidal man in the river.

When I arrived at the river, I witnessed a man in the center of the river, and I called to him. I spewed the typical, "You don't have to do this," speech and, "Your family and friends care about you."

The man appeared confused. Bystanders had gathered on the overhead bridge and were snapping pictures and videos with their cell phones.

Much to my surprise, the gentleman swam to the bank and got out. He was fully nude.

"We can get you help," I said to him.

He laughed and asked, "For what?"

I explained we had received calls that the man was suicidal, and the man appeared confused by this news as well.

"I ain't suicidal," he laughed. "I'm drunk."

The man had a few beers and decided to go skinny dipping.

Now, I'm not sure what prompted callers to report this man as suicidal. My guess is that we don't get too many people swimming in that part of the river, and witnesses probably incorrectly assumed the man wished to end his life.

I gave the man a warning for public intox and sent him on his way.

--G.W.

Ohio

■■■■■■■■■■■■■■■■■■■■■■■■■■■■■■■■■■■■■■■

Employees at an electronics store called to alert us of a 'woman on crack, who's walking around outside and yelling at customers.'

This wasn't surprising to hear, since drugs are a huge problem in our city.

When we arrived, a woman was walking in circles, and she was yelling. But it was a false alarm.

This woman was not yelling at patrons entering/exiting the store. She explained to us that she was on her way to make a purchase, when she discovered her husband had been having an affair. The two were having a heated 'discussion,' and it only appeared the woman was yelling at others because the Bluetooth device on her ear was hidden by her long hair. She was also not under the influence.

It was a pretty open and shut case, but the woman apologized and said she had been in the moment and didn't realize she had been causing such a scene to the public.

--D.B.

....

I responded to a complaint at a local theater, where an elderly man was accused of masturbating during a G-rated movie. The man was so upset by the allegations and embarrassment of being removed from the theater that he complained of chest pains and EMS was notified.

After discussing the incident with the man, he stated he had somehow dropped popcorn down his pants and was trying to get it out without going to the restroom. He told us that his grandkids lived across the country and that he routinely went to see movies they would watch so they'd have something in common they could talk about on the phone.

This 80-something-year-old man had a clean record and had never so much as received a speeding ticket. Nursing staff mentioned popcorn falling out of the man's slacks as he disrobed for his ED admission, so we left.

--K.L.

New Jersey

■■■

One 03:30 report to respond to what the elderly caller referred to as "a vicious altercation," turned out to be a group of drunk nerds having a 'battle' in the middle of a quiet side street. There was absolutely nothing 'vicious' about the men poking each other with their light saber replicas.

--X.W.

New York

<u>No Faith in Humanity</u>

Not only as an officer of the law, but also as a human being, I feel it is not my place to judge. But, because I am both, I admit I do have judgmental thoughts, especially after some of the things I've seen.

One year, I was the responding officer to our local park. We are in a suburban area and often do receive public disturbance calls to the park in question, but this call was different. A three-year-old was approaching female adults in the park, asking for help to find her mother. Three years old.

When I arrived, the child was upset, but she was the sweetest, most darling little girl I'd ever met (with exception to my own daughters, of course). She seemed to shy away from my male partner but took well to me almost instantly. We questioned the women who'd called 911, and then we questioned the toddler. She stated her mommy brought her to the park to play and told her to go swing or play on the slide. She then stated she was hungry, but when she went to tell her mommy, the adult 'disappeared.' The little girl found grown-ups to help her, but nobody could locate the child's guardian.

My partner searched the parking lot, and I walked the playground area with the child. She tried to tell me what her mother looked like, but it's hard to get a good description based off, "She's really pretty, but she's fat, too." (I do admit that the description made me chuckle.)

Furthermore, this toddler only knew her first name. She couldn't tell us anything about her father, didn't know her last name, and only seemed to know what children of that age know when identifying family members, such as 'Aunt Jane,' or

'Uncle Joe who sleeps in mommy's bed sometimes.'

About 30 minutes into looking for the child's mother, we broke down and called for someone from CPS to take custody of the child. This left our little girl in tears. I even cried because she clung to me and refused to let go. The CPS representative had to pry the little girl from me so we could continue our investigation.

We called in support patrols to search the park and interview potential witnesses. An hour in, and we still had no leads.

An adult male approached us and pointed to the restroom area. He stated there was a woman passed out on the floor, and she had a needle in her arm. He said he didn't know if she was breathing, and he didn't have a phone to call from the restroom, so he alerted us instead.

We entered the dingy restroom and, indeed, a woman was passed out on the concrete floor. She had urinated on herself. Her arm was tied off so tightly that her fingertips were turning blue. Her lips were gray and she was barely breathing.

This woman was also very pregnant.

We called for EMS transport and the patient coded during the transport. I wish I could tell you that this story ended well, but it didn't. She died, and so did the fetus she was carrying. We determined from the contents of her billfold that she was the mother of the toddler we found unattended in the park. After a good amount of time, we were finally able to track down a relative, but the relative refused to be involved in the case and wanted nothing to do with the three-year-old. That child, to my understanding, has now been in foster care for a few years now, bouncing from house to house but not having a place to call a home.

I understand addiction can consume you, make you a ghost of who you used to be, but I'm still angry about this. I'm in this line of work to protect others, and yes, most of the time it's to protect them from themselves. I cannot fathom being pregnant and shooting heroin while my toddler was playing at the park. I simply can't imagine leaving my babies alone like that.

I try so hard not to judge the people I encounter, but there are days I want to grab the guy on his 14th arrest for residential burglary, shake him, and scream at him to stop being a piece of shit. I see things that don't make sense at all, like this woman who OD'd in the bathroom. I don't know if I'm the only officer who feels this way or not, but I'm starting to lose faith that there's much good left in the world. I struggle to go home in a good mood. My children and husband keep me going. I don't know what I'd do without them. When I'm not with my family, I look around for signs of goodness in the world, but I'm seeing fewer and fewer examples that people in this world care about each other anymore.

Despite all of this, I will continue to serve my community. I took an oath to protect and serve, and I do both with pride. It's just hard not to feel like throwing in the towel and starting my own daycare business, leaving this field completely.

I do hope you share this story, just in case others out there feel the way I feel.

--M.P.

Florida

<u>Power Struggle</u>

As I write to you, I am strongly considering retiring from my department. I have been an officer for 27 years and have seen just about all there is to see. I no longer feel that I can make a difference. The world is falling apart around us, and nobody seems to mind.

I recently responded to a noise complaint. The caller stated this was a possible domestic violence incident, which we take seriously because when arriving to a domestic violence complaint, we just never know what we're going to find. A partner once responded to one such complaint, only to be shot in the neck by a drunk husband. That officer died on scene, and the shooter then put the gun in his own mouth and ended his life. The shooter's wife was in intensive care for a week before she passed away due to injuries sustained in her attack.

You NEVER know what you're going to roll up on. You must prepare yourself for the worst-case scenario at all times and act accordingly. You can only pray that your reflexes and nerves act along with your rational thoughts, but that's not always the case. Even officers panic.

I arrived at a small house on a corner lot and could hear screaming as I approached the residence. I could also hear what sounded like a power tool, but I could not see through windows at first to determine the source of the noise.

I knocked on the door three times before I walked around the house and knocked at the back door. It was there, as I was standing on the back stoop, that I could see through a window what appeared to be a pre-teen using a small chainsaw on a closed interior door. A bleeding child was crouched in the corner of the room, attempting to move behind a sofa. I forcefully entered the residence at this point, after calling for an additional unit and an ambulance.

Once inside, I ordered a young male to place the chainsaw on the ground. He looked right at me and said, "Shut the fuck up."

This subject was between the age of 11 and 14, I learned a short time later.

Again, I ordered the child to place the chainsaw on the ground. A woman was screaming from the other side of the door, pleading for her life and that of her other children's' lives. The 5-to-8-year old in the corner was crying loudly and begged the boy to 'not kill mommy.'

Attempting to speak to the pre-teen was useless. He had zero interest in talking it out. He repeatedly referred to his mother as 'the bitch,' and he said he wanted her dead. I explained I did not want to see him injured, to which he replied that he hoped I killed him so he could be famous.

At one point, the boy managed to get the chainsaw teeth through the door, and while he was focused on this, I took him down with the best tackle I could muster. We were both injured by the chainsaw before its failsafe kicked in and the device shut itself off.

With the child's mother and at least one other child screaming from the bedroom, and another injured child screaming from beside the sofa, the subject and I wrestled for what felt like ages. We both got in a few good punches to each other, before I finally disregarded that voice in my head that was telling me not to discharge my weapon against a child. I did what needed to be done, and I deployed a taser on the boy. This did not stop him from struggling and acting violently, but it did give me time to cuff him.

The subject's mother emerged from the bedroom with a toddler on her hip. This woman was bleeding from a large gash in her upper arm, and the toddler's face was bloody. I questioned the mother on what had transpired, to which she responded that she told her son that she did not have enough money to purchase the video game he wanted, and he would have to wait until her next paycheck to get the game. The boy then 'went insane.'

Upon speaking to the boy, he confirmed the events and said he was 'tired of his mom's bullshit excuses,' and if he said he wanted a video game, that meant he wanted it right now, not in two more weeks.

The boy assaulted his siblings, first punching the toddler in the face and then using a kitchen knife to slash his mother's arm while she attempted to protect her child. The boy's mother, knowing her other child was playing outside, locked herself and the toddler in a bedroom.

When the other sibling saw the pre-teen taking a chainsaw from the garage, he/she followed inside and the boy again used the knife to cut the child, who then attempted to hide.

Now, I know you didn't ask for my opinion, but I'm going to give it to you anyway.

We are living in a society that searches for fame and fortune above all else. We have become lazy, dependent on technology to not only perform for us, but also to raise our children. It is far easier to sit a child in front of a tablet or computer or phone or television that it is to listen to a child scream after you say 'no,' a word most children can't handle these days because they hear it so sparingly. We have become too strict on when to dispense consequences and too loose on expectations.

I have responded to calls of unruly children before, and I have encountered teenage thugs in the act of armed robbery or breaking and entering. I have arrested youth for drug possession or drinking underage. I understand kids will be kids, and I understand adults make mistakes, sometimes when they are in their right minds and sometimes when they are not. This call, however, was something I cannot wrap my head around. This is, or was, my breaking point. I feel that for every person I save, two hundred more criminals are out there and though we may win one battle, we are effectively losing this war. Our calls are becoming exceedingly outrageous. I don't know if I can do this anymore.

If I could give advice to anyone considering this field, let me say this. Don't you dare take this job if you're more interested in making money or being powerful or 'having it made.' Those kinds of officers are just as much part of the problem as the people we try to keep off the streets. Do follow this path if you have it in your heart to do all you can to save lives, but don't go into it thinking it's going to be sunshine and roses because most days it's anything but. There are no words for how fulfilled you will be when things go the way you want, but similarly, there will be no words for how broken you feel when things go wrong—and when things go wrong, they usually do so in a matter of seconds, that when you think about later, feel like a span of years that you tell yourself you could have done something differently to change the outcome. Maybe you could have, maybe you couldn't. Law enforcement is learning to deal with the reality that what's done is done and all you can do is move forward and try to make it better for the next family. Enter this field only if you can give it all you've got and then dig down to a reserve tank and give it even more when times get tough. That's what this field is all about.

I don't know how we, as a race, ended up where we are, but I know I'm now questioning my ability to make anything better, and I'm not so sure I have anything else to give.

--Initials and location withheld at request

While awaiting EMS, my subject (who had sustained a self-inflicted gunshot wound after he shot himself in the foot during an armed robbery) groaned and asked, "Do you think they'll give me any Morpheus on the way to the hospital?"

He did *not* receive any Morpheus (or morphine) during transport.

He *did,* however, receive an armed officer at his bedside until he was discharged and transported directly to jail.

--C.J.

Arizona

<u>Behind Bars?</u>

The dumbest criminal I've encountered was a man who tried to break in a shop after hours. When I arrived, the man had peed himself and was crying so much that I had to pull my portable oxygen tank from my trunk and let him hold the mask to his face while I called for assistance.

This idiot couldn't get through the metal security gate at the front of the building, so he walked around back, to where thick metal rods were cemented to the ground inches from each other. He was skinny, but not skinny enough to squeeze between the bars.

You guessed it. My guy was stuck between the bars. He could lift one arm, but his other arm was stuck, along with his head and legs. He was barely able to pull his cell phone out of his pocket to dial 999.

He confessed to the operator by using speakerphone because he couldn't lift that arm to his mouth to speak.

Unfortunately for the subject, it started to rain and it was already chilly. To make matters worse, most of the fire brigade was out on a call, and the only vehicle with the cutters we needed was assisting out of area. My subject was forced to remain stuck between the bars for nearly an hour, until someone arrived with the equipment we needed to cut him loose.

Not only was this man jailed, but he was also ordered to community service and was ordered to pay restitution to the shop owners.

--D.F.

U.K.

Hi-YA!

Let me tell you the story about the craziest arrest I've ever made.

It was late, well after midnight, on a weeknight. Our station received a call to the non-emergency number, and the caller stated there was a man in the park acting strangely. The female caller gave a rough detail of the man's clothes but could offer no more information because she felt afraid to continue her after-work jog and returned to her vehicle.

I was working alone that night and was dispatched to the park. It wasn't difficult to find the subject because I could hear him screaming from the pavilion I pulled up to. He was across the park, which was at least a good half a mile.

When I drove around the park and approached the man, I witnessed the nutcase doing his version of a cartwheel. Essentially, this man was throwing himself to the ground and popping out of a lopsided somersault, where he'd perform the actions all over again.

This man was in his early twenties and was a twig. He was wearing an oversized hoodie and jeans that were as tight as the leggings my wife wears. As I moved in closer, I could smell alcohol seeping from his pores.

"Care to tell me what you're doing out here so late?" I asked.

As soon as I finished my sentence, the young man pulled a weapon from his hoodie pocket. Reflexively, I drew my weapon.

It took me a second to realize what the young man was holding, but it soon became obvious: he was holding a pair of nunchucks. He then began wildly swinging the weapons and I took a step back, when it was clear the man had no idea how to properly use them. I decided to let fate take its course. I didn't have to wait too long.

"I'm a powerful ninja," the man screamed at me, as he continued swinging the weapons.

"Have you always been one, or just after a few too many drinks?" I asked with a laugh.

"I play Mortal Kombat," he replied with a stone expression.

This caused me to double over, laughing. I holstered my weapon, feeling this man was of no threat to me.

The subject apparently didn't find this funny because he started doing more cartwheel-somersault-hybrid moves and returned to swinging the nunchucks and telling me he had been declared 'the last ninja' by 'the most decorated sensei in history.'

Well, 'the last ninja' wacked himself in the testes with his nunchucks and fell to the ground. He sobbed for approximately 10-seconds before he vomited on the sidewalk and passed out.

This young man's BAC was three times the legal limit and he was admitted to the hospital for overnight observation. I was called back just as my shift was ending to speak to the young man.

You know, around here, most of our drunks exhibit embarrassment or remorse upon sobering up. This man, however, did not.

"Do you remember what happened last night?" I asked him, after introducing myself.

He stated he did not, so I explained.

His reaction?

"Well, if I didn't drink as much, I would've fucked you up."

"Is that so?" I asked with a grin.

The man didn't take so kindly to this response and leapt out of his bed. He then (weakly) 'karate-chopped' me in the neck and was subsequently arrested for assault on an officer.

What a way to end my shift!

--K.D.

Oregon

<u>Lurking in the Dark</u>

Our station is small and operated by one sheriff, two deputies, one 'official' operator (our sheriff's wife), and two volunteer deputies. We are mainly active during the day, and I think we've maybe had five or six night calls over the course of a year, so whichever one of us gets stuck on the night shift mostly sleeps and only gets up in case the phone rings. Our town's population is under 200, and most of our citizens are elderly. We live in a quiet, rural location and enjoy every minute of it.

One night, when our sheriff was out of town on a hunting trip, his wife called my cell phone eight times in two minutes. I was groggy when I answered on her ninth attempt to reach me; it was 11 PM and well past my bedtime.

When I answered, I could hear Jane screaming. I heard her mention she was at the station. I couldn't catch anything else she was saying because she was so frantic. Then, the line went dead.

Thinking something terrible had occurred, I threw on a pair of overalls over my pajamas, slipped on flip flops, and grabbed my .45 out of the closet. I told my wife to call our other guys and have them meet me at the station to check on Jane.

The ride to 'town' took about five minutes. My pickup was fishtailing down the gravel roads and I'm sure I was going at least 75 MPH down most of those roads, if not faster.

When I pulled into the station lot, I could see Jane's car, but I couldn't see her. None of the lights were on in the station. Something was wrong.

I got out of my truck and attempted to enter the station, but I was locked out. I called out to Jane, but all I could hear was silence. I left my station keys at home and was S.O.L until the other guys arrived with their keys.

With my firearm in one hand and my phone as a flashlight in the other, I crept around the building, hoping the back was open.

"Jane?" I called again.

I heard Jane scream from a short distance and I yelled into the dark, "Where are you? Are you hurt?"

"Help me!" she hollered.

I ran toward her voice.

"Don't get too close," she warned. "They'll attack."

"Huh?" I asked. "Coyotes?"

"No," she said. I could tell she was crying, but I still couldn't see what was going on.

I'd like to think I'm a man of realistic and rational thoughts, but at that moment, I don't know what I was expecting to see in the dark.

I extended my cell phone as far as my arm would reach, hoping to get a peek at what 'they' were. As I cautiously inched closer to Jane's voice, the light of my phone caught at least 12 roosters and hens pecking around the base of a tree.

"Make them go away," Jane pleaded.

I looked up to the medium-size tree, and there was Jane, hugging a large limb and barely perched on a slender branch under her feet.

"What in the hell are you doing in the tree?" I asked. "I thought you were being attacked or something."

She said, "I was!"

"Well, get on down here," I told her.

I tried to approach the tree to help Jane down, but the birds had something else in mind. They started chasing me, flopping around in a huff, pecking at my legs and bare toes. I tried to lightly kick at the flock, but this ticked them off even more. I'm still not sure what had them so riled up or how they got out of the nearest neighbor's roost.

Our salaried deputies showed up around the same time and our solution to the bird problem was to scatter one of those snack-sized bags of cheddar popcorn from the gas station on the ground so we could move Jane down from the tree.

We found Jane's cell phone on the ground, broken. She told us one of our volunteer deputies had to leave early, so she went in to man the phones, but she'd locked her keys in the car and couldn't get in the station or her car to seek refuge from the 'killer' birds.

"That was the only place to go," she explained, motioning to the tree.

Once we all calmed down, we had a good laugh, but damn if that wasn't one of the scariest moments in my life.

We still give Jane crap about it, and her husband won't let her live it down.

--T.S.

Texas

Man's Best Friend

I responded to a report of a man dealing drugs near a high school.

Of course, as soon as I parked and stepped out of my vehicle, the subject bolted.

I engaged in a foot pursuit for approximately two blocks, chasing a man in his mid-30s and a large-breed dog that ran beside him.

When I finally caught the subject, I said, "You're acting pretty guilty for someone I haven't even accused yet."

"Whatever it is, I didn't do it," he said.

I motioned to the sidewalk, where baggies of heroin had fallen out during the chase.

"The evidence literally leads to you," I countered.

"Man," he protested, "I don't have anything on me. You can't arrest me if I'm not holding."

I looked to the man's dog, who'd taken a seated position next to his owner. The dog was fitted with a miniature backpack printed with the Superman logo. The backpack was partially unzipped and heroin baggies were sticking out.

The long-story-short lesson here is this: Yes, you *can* get arrested for possession, even if your dog is the one wearing the backpack that contains your supply.

--Initials and location withheld at request

Tip from an arresting officer:

If you are going to rob a gas station, pick a costume that hides your face, too. Dressing up as a Twister game mat does nothing to hide your identity, if you leave your face exposed.

Once in custody, the dipshit told us he thought the cashier would be distracted by the costume so much that she wouldn't remember his face.

Maybe so, but the security cameras weren't distracted.

Moron.

--D.W.

Location unknown

<u>Indecent Exposure</u>

It is my opinion that LEOs have the best stories about public nudity. Their stories sure seem to beat even the wildest college stories. Here are a few:

My partner and I responded to complaints of a nude man disturbing the peace.

When we arrived at the **dog park**, we instantly spotted the naked individual. He was running alongside the fence (with his balls and penis flopping in the wind), yelling for excited dogs to play with him while the dogs' owners attempted to keep the animals far away from the subject.

I completely lost my professionalism when this middle-age man turned around and defecated in front of us and about 20 other people watching from inside the dog park.

While we were arresting the man for disorderly conduct and exposing himself, he asked me if I wanted to have sex with him. I declined and told him my husband probably wouldn't appreciate that very much.

We transported the man to the ER, where we learned he was under the influence of PCP and alcohol. Shocker.

--O.N.

Maine
▪▪▪

I'll never forget this. Back when I was a rookie to our department, I was sent across town to a complaint from the Reverend's wife. She had arrived at church early that Sunday to prepare for a group of baptisms that would take place prior to the weekly sermon. When she arrived, she found a naked woman ducking between the pews.

I was excited to be the responding officer because it was my first 'real' complaint, besides traffic stops and domestic complaints between neighbors.

When I arrived, the Reverend's wife was standing outside the church's side entrance. Her face was beet red and she looked embarrassed more than anything else.

"She's defiling our church," she croaked.

"She probably had too much to drink and somehow ended up in here during the night," I said.

"No," said the Reverend's wife, gripping my arm. "She is *defiling our church.* She's…pleasuring herself in there. I couldn't be in there while she was doing that."

Well, I was even more excited to go inside because this was going to make one heck of a story to tell the guys back at the station.

When I entered the church, there was a woman pleasuring herself with a taper candlestick. What was more disturbing about this was that the woman had injured herself while performing this action, and there was blood all over the floor. I couldn't find her clothes anyplace, so I borrowed a pea coat from the coat closet after I cuffed her, and I draped the coat over the woman. She screamed the entire time, including as I walked her to my squad car. It was clear there was something 'off' about this woman.

Back in the day, mental health was a taboo subject, so we didn't mention the incident outside of the station. That incident made me grow up and grow out of my 'excited for action' stage because it exposed me to the reality of the job. If I remember correctly, the woman was sent to a hospital and then transferred to a group home for the mentally ill. I do recall quite clearly that all church services that week were canceled with limited explanation to parishioners as to why.

--W.J.

Connecticut

■■■

I responded to a report of a man exposing himself to shoppers at a busy grocery store. Clerks had driven the man out of the store, but a group of teenagers in the parking lot flagged me down and pointed me in the right direction.

I found the man wearing only a sleeveless shirt and a pair of Crocs shoes. I have no idea where his pants were. He was masturbating himself in a vehicle's tailpipe.

This sick individual was arrested and convicted on several charges. I'd always heard of people doing things like this, but this was the first (and only) time I'd encountered it.

--R.J.

Washington

■■■■■■■■■■■■■■■■■■■■■■■■■■■■■■■■■■■■■■

Someone in the neighborhood requested officers to conduct a welfare check on two small children who were found wandering the area unattended. When we visited the home, I was completely shocked that the mother of the small children answered the door in the nude. She stepped out on the porch to speak with me, and she didn't seem to mind that she didn't have clothes on and was exposing herself to all her watching neighbors.

She was placed under arrest when she said the magic words: "Wanna come do a line [of cocaine] with me?"

--B.L.

California
■■

Several drivers called 911 to report a motorcyclist was speeding down the interstate with a naked woman as his passenger. I was positioned a few miles ahead of the route that was reported and waited for him to pass me.

Yep, as he flew by, I could clearly see a nude female passenger seated behind him. Her hair was blowing in the wind.

When I pulled the motorcyclist over, I quickly discovered his passenger was not alive. The man was transporting a realistic sex mannequin. He stated the adult store clerk attempted to sell him clothes for the doll (which was a sort of firm silicone, I believe; it was not inflatable), but he told me, "There's kind of no point, you know? I'm not gonna use her while she's wearing clothes."

I didn't know how to respond, so when the driver told me he lived five miles away, I let him off with a warning for speeding and suggested he put some clothes on his 'woman' if he transported her again.

The driver thanked me for not citing him and told me the only place he'd be moving the doll was to and from his closet/bed. Uh…okay.

I felt weird about telling him to have a good day because I had an idea about what he was going to do when he arrived at his home, so I just told him to be careful and slow down.

--I.G.

North Carolina

My first solo run ever was to a busy hotel. We had received several calls of a woman passed out in the hallway of an upper floor.

What dispatch neglected to tell me is that the woman was naked.

She was also covered in butter.

I have no idea what lead to either, but she was transported by EMS to the ER and was admitted to ICU for an overdose.

--K.C.

Nevada
■■

I am a 911 dispatcher. I live alone and have four cats who often run wild through my home and create quite the ruckus.

One night, I was playing an online video game and was wearing a headset. (You would think that I would hate wearing head gear outside of the office, but I actually enjoy speaking to strangers, so I guess my job fits me like a glove.) Between the sounds of my game, I heard some thumping, but I didn't think that was unusual because my cats climb up their carpeted tower and jump down to the hardwood floor. With four cats, this can become quite loud, so I just brushed off the noise.

I was waiting in the game 'lobby' to enter a scenario and had just enough time to use the restroom and grab a soda from the fridge.

When I entered my bathroom, there was a naked man standing in my shower! The water wasn't on, he didn't say anything, and there were no clothes in sight.

I ran out of my house so fast that I didn't even close the door behind me. My neighbor called the cops, but by the time they arrived, the naked man was gone.

Unfortunately, three of my four cats escaped from the house during this, and it took two days to track them down and bring them back inside.

I don't exactly know how the naked man got in the house (I was told the lock was installed slightly crooked and the intruder possibly jiggled the door and handle enough until he gained entry, which would explain the noise I heard), and I don't know why he was naked. Officers never found him.

I called a repairman to replace the locks on all my doors and I installed security cameras around all entrances.

--D.W.

Arizona

__Not the Brightest Bunch__

We received a call of a Facebook sale gone wrong. According to the female caller, she had posted an ad to sell an Xbox for $100.

The caller then stated she received a message from a male who stated he did not have cash, but he wanted to know if she would like to trade the Xbox for meth. She told us that she agreed to this trade.

(Yep. Yep. Stay with me, now.)

This woman explained that she met the man at a strip club to complete the transaction, and all seemed to go well. She gave him the Xbox, and he gave her the meth.

Then, she explained that she entered the strip club and shot up in the bathroom, but she did not get high.

Yes, you got it…The caller was hoping to file a complaint that she was 'ripped off' by the male who gave her bad drugs. She gave us the man's Facebook contact information, and we realized we were already in contact with this man.

See, earlier that day, another officer took a phone call that told a slightly less incriminating story.

The male caller stated that he purchased an electronic device from a woman for $100. He stated that when he got home and attempted to use the device, it wouldn't work. He told us that he took the device apart to see if this was a problem he could fix, but he said most of the device's components had been removed and the device was reassembled. He wanted us to mandate a refund for the device, although there wasn't a whole lot we could do with the information we had.

You're reading all of this correctly.

We staged a meet with both parties at a public location because neither wanted to come to the station. We arrested both for their illegal activities. Both were charged for possession of meth when confronted.

I wish all our arrests were that easy.

--J.L.

Indiana

YES, you CAN still be cited for using your cell phone while operating a motor vehicle, even if you're using Snapchat instead of texting or calling someone.

#DUH.

--L.B.

Virginia

Playlist

My partner and I responded to a noise complaint at an outdoor celebration and tried to give the partygoers every chance in the world to comply with our requests to turn down the volume to their music.

One rowdy gentleman approached me and said, "Hey, hold my beer real quick. I have your answer."

The man then swiped through his iPod until the song 'Fuck the Police' came on. He turned up the volume on his stereo system.

My partner connected his phone to the aux cord in our patrol car as we were transporting the man to jail. We played 'I Fought the Law (And the Law Won)' on repeat.

Let's take a look at the scorecard one more time:

Police: 1

Arrested Subject: 0

--R.G.

Ohio

This isn't the Hilton

One of our inmates was awaiting extradition to another state on charges of rape and molestation of minors. He had been with us approximately two weeks and had another two weeks before someone from the out-of-state facility would arrive for his transport.

This inmate requested a lawyer with a week to go at our facility.

No joke, this inmate attempted to sue our facility for failing to provide brunch options or desserts, stated he felt it was unfair that our bedding had such a low thread count, and he said he was refused his right to smoke.

His case was (rightfully) tossed out by a judge, but we were advised to 'tiptoe' around him for the duration of his stay. I found the entire situation to be ridiculous. Your stay in jail is NOT supposed to feel as luxurious as a stay at a five-star hotel!

--S.V.

South Carolina

Bait

Our department decided to make a post in a Facebook group that was created for people in our community to complain about everything and anything.

The post, which we thought was funny and something that nobody would fall for, read, 'Found: two bags of heroin. Call (our station's number) if you are missing from your supply. We will set up a meeting to return your heroin if you can provide proof that it belongs to you.'

FOUR subjects contacted us about this 'found' heroin and agreed to meet us in front of the fire station. Three of the subjects brought syringes and/or drugs as proof that the drugs belonged to them, and the fourth brought hospital discharge papers proving he/she had overdosed recently and received Narcan.

All four individuals were arrested.

When we made the post, we had no idea that anyone would take it seriously.

--Initials and location withheld at request

<u>Obey First Responders!</u>

This is a personal account of something I witnessed this month, and I'm still frustrated about what occurred.

After a toss-and-turn night of two hours of sleep, I woke at the crack of dawn to my dogs barking and someone shouting outside. My first reaction, since I am such a cheerful morning person, was to express anger in form of spewing a long line of curse words. I honestly thought someone high on drugs was outside.

When I let my dogs in the backyard, a neighbor rushed to my fence and asked, "Did you hear that explosion? The whole place is on fire!"

"What place?" I asked. "I didn't hear an explosion, but I heard someone yell."

"Yeah, there was a guy trying to warn everyone in the connected business to get out and move their cars away from the building."

I walked to the front yard and took a quick peek at the commotion as a fleet of fire trucks, police cars, and ambulances arrived on scene. A business across the street from my home was up in flames.

I returned inside and continued about my business. My writing area is right next to a window that faces the street and the affected business, and I could see all personal and business vehicles had been moved to side streets. Some were even parked in neighbors' yards to make room for more first responders. I could see injured employees being transported to ambulances, and the amount of police presence was amazing. Adjacent counties sent fire crews to work with our county's crews, and city officials arrived shortly after to mark the road as closed. Officers parked their vehicles at every road leading to mine and blocked off the area for two blocks in each direction.

My friends began sending me messages and tagging me in Facebook posts about the fire, as it was unclear just what was on fire in the area. People were reporting that they could see smoke all the way across town.

As first responders tended to injured parties and crews scrambled to extinguish the fire, curious bystanders began swarming the block. I even witnessed three adults place folding lawn chairs on my front lawn so they could watch the action live. There were people I recognized from living five blocks away, right there in front of my house, using their cell phones to record videos and take pictures. Frustrated first responders repeatedly asked these people to leave the area, and the crews explained the fire was unpredictable and the business housed volatile chemicals that could explode at any moment. This was such a serious concern that crews were considering evacuating surrounding residents.

Some bystanders listened to authorities, but others stuck around. Officers did nothing about this because their priorities were all about tending to the injured and getting the fire put out as soon as possible.

An hour into the battle, bystanders were still flooding in. Law enforcement took to Facebook to plead with the public not to visit the scene. Few listened.

Shortly after law enforcement posted the warning for citizens to stay clear of the area, I heard a series of explosions and looked up.

Chemicals stored in the building had exploded and acted as accelerants. Two bystanders who were standing close enough to the fire to reach out and touch it were injured. Both were severely burned.

What I found even more shocking than that, was how other gawkers reacted.

People were still taking videos and pictures. My social media home screen refreshed and there were pictures being posted online by the same people who were standing in my yard and lining up on sidewalks up and down the block.

As readers of this series and my previous, you know all too well the importance of listening and obeying law enforcement and first responders. Unfortunately, many do not understand that these first responders are not attempting to hide information from the public, but instead are attempting to protect the public.

On the day of the fire, first responders knew better than anyone else watching the scene exactly what type of chemicals were inside the building and how those chemicals would potentially react. These emergency personnel are trained professionals, so it's especially frustrating to know others refuse to listen for the sake of the drama.

Ignoring orders from authorities resulted in one patient in rough condition and one person being flown by helicopter to a hospital three- hours away.

Please, please…If a first responder asks you to do something, please do not assume he/she is asking for no reason. Complying might just save your life.

Obnoxious

We had been searching for a wanted man for several months. He was wanted for forced entrance/armed residential burglary (while residents were home), battery (on a man in his 90s), sexual assault (on a woman in her 90s), auto theft, and the list goes on. We knew what the guy looked like; he was caught on security cameras not only at the home he burglarized, but also at the gas station (while driving a stolen vehicle). At the gas station, he decided to use stolen credit cards to pay at the pump, and then proceeded to rob the convenience store clerk at gunpoint. He shot a clerk in the process. (Don't worry, that clerk lived.)

This was one bad man, the lowest of the low.

To make matters worse, this guy was also cocky as all get-out. There were times he'd call us once a day, or there were times he'd call once a week. Each time, he would call from a 'burner' cell phone, which is a disposable cell phone that he did not keep in his possession for a long time. This made it difficult to track him. He seemed to derive great pleasure from taunting us. He usually boasted we would never catch him. Sometimes he would call and go on insane rants, like how he went on a curse-filled tirade about something that happened in the media. (One example of this was a 10-minute-long rant about an arrest story that had gone viral.)

Occasionally, he would threaten our staff. He once told our operator that he would enter her apartment while she was sleeping, rape and murder her, and kidnap her young daughter to keep as his sex slave. Our operator understood that this man was deranged and liked to get a rise out of people, but the next time he called, he gave explicit details about our operator's day of running errands after her shift ended. He was close enough to us that he'd been following her. We posted officers outside her apartment building for weeks, but the fugitive never came around.

Finally, FINALLY, we received a phone call from a waitress who stated the subject was in her restaurant. We sent in officers in plain-clothes first, as to not cause a scene. These officers felt there was no safe time during the man's dining experience to approach him, so we waited until he exited the building and nabbed him as he was attempting to break into a car in the lot.

This man did not go down without a fight. Luckily, he was not carrying a weapon that day. I've thanked God every morning since then that he wasn't, because that encounter could have gone so many different ways. We did use force on the subject, as he threw several punches at officers. Eventually, we managed to pin and cuff him.

I was the officer responsible for reading this subject his rights. While I was doing so, he attempted to run twice, and he wouldn't shut his damn mouth. He started off by talking over me. I started from the beginning several times. I wanted this to be a clean, solid arrest.

Then, the man began doing what small children do, singing 'la, la, la' loudly.

He refused to acknowledge his rights or anything else I said to him.

We booked the subject in a solitary cell. There was no way he was facing anything less than a five-year sentence. There was just no way, not with all the charges he had and evidence we had.

The son of a bitch waited until the next day to request an attorney, and he filed a complaint stating I failed to administer his rights fully, and that he did not understand his rights. He stated I stuttered and paused throughout reading his rights, and that I stopped and started over several times. Not only that, but the subject's attorney alleged that I had improperly persuaded the subject to confess to crimes without an attorney present.

(The only way I could even see that as a possibility is when the man bragged about a crime, and I responded, "Just like you hit that house over on ABC Lane and terrorized that family, huh?" I admit, I should have remained quiet, but apparently because the subject laughed and said, "Yeah," it became a pressured admission of guilt.)

The subject then told his attorney that he felt 'victimized' by me and requested a restraining order. I was suspended with pay, pending the ruling of the court. This was done as a precautionary measure.

Surely, I thought, this would be wrapped up and the guy's claims would be considered ludicrous.

Deliberation went on for a nerve-racking week and a half. Every aspect of my behavior, of my tone of voice, the volume of my voice, how I handled the subject physically…it was all scrutinized by some crooked lawyer looking for an easy paycheck—and let's face it, when one of his clients ran with the charges that our subject had, there was no bullshitting anyone and saying that this was for more anything more than money. Everyone could see our subject was guilty. We had undeniable video evidence of the subject shooting the owner of a car he was stealing. We had witness testimony from the homeowners he assaulted. We had fingerprints. We had voice recordings.

I didn't sleep for that entire week and a half because I was so terrified that we were going to lose and this ass was going to skate.

Luckily, after being presented the allegations and facts, a judge ruled in our station's favor and said our behavior was acceptable and legal. Thankfully, the subject did not file an appeal against the ruling.

This guy's still locked up and should be behind bars for much of the rest of his natural life. And I'm grateful for that every single day.

--Initials and location withheld at request

<u>Danger, Danger</u>

My most memorable 911 call was as follows (to the best of my recollection):

Me: 911, what's your emergency?

Caller: Uh, hey. So, I have a problem.

Me: What seems to be the problem, sir?

Caller: Well, I just bought this house in an auction, and there's some stuff I don't really want. I need to get rid of it, but I don't know what to do.

Me: Sir, this is line is restricted for emergencies only. May I suggest calling 411 to contact a disposal company?

Caller: No, you don't understand. This is an emergency. I don't know what to do with it. I got a fridge and a freezer and a barrel down in the root cellar, and I need to get rid of these things right now. Like, I mean it. I need to get rid of this stuff now.

Me: Sir, do you understand you can face charges for abusing an emergency line? I need to have an open line, in case someone with a real emergency needs medical or police assistance.

Caller: But this *is* an emergency.

Me, losing my cool: Okay. You know what? Let me just get your contact information, and I will send an officer to your location because your definition of an emergency is winning an old refrigerator in a real estate auction.

Caller: Well, you should make sure they send those guys with the boxes to blow stuff up, like they have in the movies.

Me: What?

Caller: Yeah, that's what I've been trying to tell you. The whole fridge and barrel and freezer—they have, like, tons of dynamite in them.

(You should LEAD with that kind of information, by the way.)

Me: Come again?

Caller: Yeah, dynamite. But I didn't touch it because I saw that episode of *Lost* where that science guy was talking and got blown to pieces when that stick he was holding blew up. I ain't dumb, you know.

Me: Sir, is this a prank call?

Caller: Huh? No! I need to get rid of this stuff before the whole house goes up. I paid ten-grand for this house, and I'm not losing that investment. Figured I can flip it and still come out with a good thirty-grand when it's all said and done.

Me: And there's really dynamite in your root cellar?

Caller: Yeah. That's what I've been trying to tell you.

Me: And how much would you say is down there?

Caller: I don't know. I think, maybe, like ten sticks in each thing. But the barrel might not have that many. I didn't see more, but there were a lot of places I didn't look. Like, there are some old crates down there. Lots of weird weapon-things, too.

Me: Weapons?

Caller: Yep. Bunch of metal things to hit people with.

Me: Like a mace?

Caller: I guess that's what you call them.

Me: Sir, I need you to move as far away from the house as possible. Is anyone else in the home with you?

Caller: No. And I'm already outside. I'm on the back porch.

Me: I'm sending a response team.

The caller's newly-purchased home had been condemned, after being vacant for decades. We learned the home was originally owned by a wealthy man who co-owned a coal mine in the early-1900s. We have no idea how the dynamite (32 sticks were found) ended up stored in the furniture/appliances left in the root cellar or why the last owner did not notify authorities of the dynamite. We're also not sure why the dynamite never exploded, but we've since deemed it as fate for the new owner and the community. The 'weapons to hit people with' were old hammers and mining picks.

--D.P.

West Virginia

Inconvenienced

Your stories about impatient ER patients resonated with me, because as an officer, I also face my fair share of people who act like me doing my job is the worst possible thing that could ever happen to them. One particular incident stands out in my mind.

On the outskirts of town, we have a two-lane highway that is heavily-trafficked. This not the only way in or out of town, but it is the preferred way by most of our townspeople and truck drivers.

One night, following a horrendous MVA that had already taken the lives of three and had left glass, blood, and chunks of metal scattered on both lanes and in the ditches, we placed officers to the north and south, blocking the highway from travelers.

I was responsible for meeting drivers on the south end of the highway. I instructed drivers to turn around and use the interstate for travel. Many expressed concerns for the MVA victims and left with no argument.

Not everyone behaves so civilly, as you are aware.

An expensive luxury sedan was approaching at lightning speed and its driver slammed on the brakes as soon I became visible.

I approached the vehicle and a woman rolled down her window.

"Sorry, ma'am, but this road is temporarily closed. There's been an accident, so we're rerouting traffic to the interstate."

"Uh, no, that's not acceptable," she said snidely.

I chuckled with disbelief. "Well, as I said, there's been an accident. This road won't be open for another few hours, at least."

"I am *not* turning around. I can get to the mall in an hour if I go this way. The interstate takes me all the way around and adds an extra twenty minutes."

"Ma'am, this road is closed. There's been an ac—."

"I heard you the first time," she shouted. "I don't care who wrecked or why. I care about getting to the mall without going out of my way."

"Ma'am, while you're concerned about a shopping trip, families have lost relatives tonight. It was a bad accident."

"Well, if they're dead, they won't care if I drive by."

"This road is closed. You need to turn around."

This woman began cussing and ranting and raving, but she finally turned around.

The audacity she had to complain about an extra twenty minutes while we were waiting for a medical team to arrive with a helicopter to fly out MVA victims clinging to dear life left me so angry that I was trembling. I'm sure none of the deceased would have complained one bit about an extra twenty minutes if they knew they could have kept their lives, saw their children and grandchildren one more time, played fetch with their dogs just one last time.

I didn't take this job so I could heckle the innocent public and ruin days. I didn't take this job so I could piss people off when I gave them a warning to slow their asses down so their cars wouldn't end up wrapped around a tree. I try to understand that people take my warnings personally, but the truth is that I took this job because I want to keep people safe, and I'm sorry that closing a road after an accident with fatalities is such a big damn inconvenience to travelers.

I do hope there are more people out there who understand I do my job with the best of intentions than those who think I wake up every morning with the sole purpose of 'meeting a quota' or 'writing a ticket for every little thing.'

--J.Y.

Tennessee

Excuses

I'm sure every officer out there has a long list of excuses they've been fed by speeders, intoxicated operators, and/or reckless drivers. Here are a few LEOs have shared with me:

- "Well, my wife would be able to tell I've been drinking if I called for a taxi. She can't tell if I drive myself."

- "Someone set my cat on fire." During the escort to the veterinarian's office to confirm the driver's pet was in distress, the driver took an unexpected left turn and we engaged in a high-speed pursuit. I lost the vehicle and never found the driver.

- I stopped a man for doing 95 in a 55. What's worse was he had two children in the car. He said his daughter had started her menstrual cycle for the first time, so he was driving to his wife's work so she could 'take care of it.' His daughter started crying and said, "Dad, I can't believe you're telling everyone. Shut up!" I gave the guy a warning.

- "McDonald's stops serving breakfast in eight minutes. Come on, lady. Give me a break." I was going to give him a break until he motioned to my pudge and added, "It looks like you like to eat. You probably love McDonald's."

- "I just found out I have Herpes and was arguing with my girlfriend about her telling my wife." That was the driver's excuse for veering off the road and hitting a mailbox.

- "Dude, relax. I have the high score on [a car racing arcade game in the Wal Mart foyer]." The teenager received his first speeding ticket that day, along with a citation for improper lane usage.

- "You're telling me it was fine for the government to draft me and send me to Vietnam, but that same government is telling me it's too dangerous to drive more than 55 MPH?" Charges: DUI, speeding, driving without a valid license, and no brake lights.

- "It's about to rain and I just got a perm."

- "My boss just got fired for stealing and I want to see her walked out by security."

- "I'm in labor," said the highly-intoxicated 49-year-old male who failed his field sobriety test.

- The highlight of my patrol career was pulling over a DeLorean for speeding. The driver used the movie quote about reaching 88 MPH. He was coming back from a car convention, and I couldn't even bring myself to ticket him because the vehicle so enamored me. He let me sit in the driver's seat and he took a picture for me.

Well, Dog-Gone

I once pulled over a woman for misusing the carpool lane.

"But I have multiple passengers," she said.

I looked to the Irish Wolfhound in the passenger seat, and three Golden Retrievers in the back kind of looked at me like they were waiting for a response. I saw a mesh bag on the floorboard that was filled with tennis balls and latex squeaky toys.

"Ma'am, you have to have human passengers."

"Can't you let slide?" she begged. "I'm gonna be late getting them to daycare."

It was hard to write her a ticket with four dogs staring at me like children do, so I let her off with a warning.

--M.M.

California

<u>Genius</u>

I responded to reports about a loud man skateboarding in an empty tennis court area behind an apartment complex.

When I arrived on scene, it was clear the man had been drinking. My first clue was that the man naked. The second clue was he reeked of alcohol.

"Sir," I asked, as I approached him, "have you been drinking tonight?"

He shrugged. "A little."

"How much would you say you've had to drink?"

He thought. "Well, maybe about ten shots."

"Ten shots?" I asked.

"And beer. I had beer, too. And then, like, two gin and tonics."

"Ah," I nodded.

"Yeah," he said. "So, like, a lot to drink."

"Uh-huh."

I motioned to the skateboard in his hand. "Any reason you're out here at two in the morning?"

"Skating's fun."

"Any reason you're naked?" I asked.

He looked down the front portion of his body with a shocked expression and said, "How 'bout that?"

"You don't remember removing your clothes?"

He shook his head. "I was passed out for a while, but then I woke up and drank some Smart Water."

"You could probably get your money back," I said under my breath.

"What?"

"I said we should probably get you back home," I told him.

I had been responding to shootings and domestic violence complaints all night, so this call was a piece of cake. I figured the guy wasn't really causing any harm, but he also didn't need to be exposing himself to half of the city, either. I gave him a ride to his mother's house across town and went right on back to dealing with the nitty gritty calls.

--E.C.

Illinois

We all have that coworker who's a few colors short of a rainbow.

During a press conference regarding a series of breaking and entering, a reporter asked, "How did the suspect gain access to the facility?"

The deputy, with a confused expression, stated, "Well, he used the handle to open the door."

He's now banned from giving interviews.

--U.R.

South Carolina

<u>Refreshing</u>

A few years ago, we had a local we all knew too well. She was always on our radar and was in and out of our jail due to drug usage. We would have liked to have seen her incarcerated to force her into sobriety, but our D.A. kept making deals with this woman that kept her out of prison. Her behavior became wildly bizarre over time, as she developed a tolerance to drugs and needed more each time to reach a high.

I was called to a convenience store during the lunch rush hour. The parking lot was packed tighter than a sardine can.

Some patrons were standing outside the convenience store, excitedly chattering between themselves. Even more were inside, gathered in a corner. I wasn't sure what I was about to encounter, because dispatch only told me there was a 'disturbance' involving this local woman.

When I went inside, a cashier rushed over to me and could hardly speak through panting. "I told her to stop. I don't even know what she's doing. Everyone started watching. We tried to stop her, but then she started throwing stuff, and nobody wanted to touch her. I didn't know what to do."

I moved to the back corner of the store, stepping over pushed-over shelves, and stepping on packages of cookies and potato chips. I ordered onlookers out of the way, but I still had to push through the crowd.

Jane was squatting on the floor in front of the beverage cooler, and I can only describe the scene as 'really freaking weird.' She was naked from the waist down. She didn't even have shoes or socks on.

This woman shook a 20-ounce bottle of Coca Cola, placed the bottle between her legs, and as soon as she removed the cap from the pop, she shoved the erupting beverage into her vagina, essentially giving herself a 'soda pop douche.' According to onlookers, this was the third pop she used to do this. Based on her expression and reaction, I would say she was experiencing sexual pleasure from this practice.

Making arrest was anything but easy. This woman and I wrestled for several minutes before she managed to get away, and then I chased her around the store for a few minutes more. All the while, patrons were coming and going. Some walked in, paid for gas, and left, just like nothing was happening or the store was a disaster. Others watched. One woman stepped over me as I was lying on the floor (I took a fall), selected candy from an endcap, and returned to the register, where the flustered clerk was trying to maintain some sense of normalcy.

I finally managed to capture and cuff my subject, but she refused to budge. I had to call for backup just to get her moved out of the building.

I thought it was all over, as we were driving toward the emergency room for a wellness exam prior to arrest, but I'm never that lucky. The subject defecated in the backseat and then rolled in it, smearing crap all over herself and my unit.

Lab results showed she had heroin and meth in her system, as well as trace amounts of cocaine.

Thankfully, no deals were made this time, and the woman was sentenced to a year in the DOC.

--T.H.

Wyoming

129

Here Piggy, Piggy, Piggy

We had an ongoing complaint from a farmer that we still talk about ten years later.

'Joe' called us one morning to let us know some hooligan had trespassed on his property. He knew this because three of his sows were wearing string bikinis and "unless they've been ordering from Frederick's of Hollywood, they didn't do it to themselves."

We didn't bother taking a report because it was a complaint that had us in stitches, and no harm was done.

Over the course of a month, Joe made six more reports. He would wake up and find his sows wearing dresses, jackets, and one morning discovered two sows had tiny sombreros tied to their heads. He seemed aggravated with each complaint, but he was irate when making his last complaint. A sow had been fitted with overalls and lost mobility. The sow was found stuck on her side, struggling to move upright.

We monitored the property overnight for a week but didn't catch anyone trespassing. We think our presence scared away the pig-dresser because Joe didn't have any more trouble.

--J.D.

Kentucky

Guys on scene played 'rock, paper, scissors' to figure out who would have the honor of transporting our perp to jail. After leading us on a lengthy foot chase, he was found hiding in an old outhouse…submerged in excrement up to his chin.

I unrolled about eight heavy-duty contractor's trash bags and lined the back of my unit. We drove with the windows rolled down, but it didn't make much of a difference. My car reeked for weeks.

--E.C.

Nebraska

<u>Poor Kid</u>

We collaborated with our local fire department and medical transport department to host a family fun night at our local park, where we manned game booths, offered free food, and even had a few rides set up for the kids.

I was approached by an older woman, who was tightly gripping a small boy's hand. The child was sobbing so hard he could hardly breathe. The woman was holding a soda can.

"What's wrong?" I asked, thinking the worst.

The woman shoved the boy forward. "Tell him what you did."

He avoided making eye contact with me and sniffled.

"Tell him," the woman repeated. "Tell him how you've been a bad boy."

The boy cried, "I stole a soda."

"You stole a soda?" I asked. I was confused. "Son, where'd you get the soda from?"

He started sobbing again.

"Answer the policeman," ordered the woman.

The boy turned and pointed to the refreshment table across the way.

I smiled. "Son, those sodas are free. You didn't steal it."

"He didn't steal it?" the old woman asked, shocked.

I shook my head. "Nope. The only food that's not free is the snack food from the EMS bake sale."

The woman was embarrassed that she had pulled this kid through the ringer, and I felt so bad for the kid that I got a couple of buddies together from fire and rescue, who made the kid an honorary fireman for the day.

--P.R.

Michigan

<u>Wow</u>

Sometimes the law sets itself up and hurts offenders in an attempt to go easy.

We had this woman who was no stranger to our officers. She was banned from many of the stores in town because she had sticky fingers. She'd been in and out of court more than twenty times in less than a year, and each time the judge would let her go with a mild reprimand. One time she stole two cars in one night and got sentenced to two days in jail. The night she was released, she went 'shopping' and stole $600 worth of makeup and clothes from a department store. She ended up back in court for that and was sentenced to community service. She still had community service she was ordered to complete from months back that she hadn't worked towards, so we were positive she wouldn't bother this time around.

We picked up this lady after we received a complaint from a liquor store attendant. The woman stole one 'fun' bottle of Captain Morgan, valued at approximately $1.50. She was identified by the clerk, was caught on security footage, and had the bottle on her person when we found her walking the streets.

I don't know if the judge was having a bad day or just finally reached the conclusion that this woman's crime spree wouldn't end, but he blew up in court and told her he was tired of seeing her day in and day out. He gave her the maximum sentence and finally enforced her probation violations. She was sentenced to prison for 18 months.

It blows my mind, it really does, that practically nothing happened when she was charged with public intox, auto theft, retail theft in excess of $500, was banned from stores in town, and had such a lengthy rap sheet and bad reputation, yet she finally went away for a year and a half to prison for stealing about a shot or two of alcohol.

I do hope the best for this woman. I hope she gets out and decides to change her life around.

But, if she doesn't, we'll be there.

--O.F.

Georgia

Lights, Camera, Action

Not only were we alerted by the alarm company, but residents near the boutique called in to report a group of men had busted out a display window and were stealing.

Three patrol cars arrived and we found four men, aging from 18-24, casually removing merchandise from the store and loading it into a pickup. A fifth man was holding a camcorder, recording his friends.

"Stop what you're doing and raise your hands," my partner demanded.

None of the men followed the order. One or two looked concerned, but they continued packing up the pickup and one guy even returned to the boutique to steal more merchandise.

"Stop what you're doing and raise your hands right now," my partner repeated.

The cameraman turned to record us and said with a laugh, "You can't arrest us. We're making a movie."

"You're stealing," my partner said.

"Well, yeah, but it's for a movie, so you can't do anything about it."

I laughed. "How do you figure?"

"Because I just told you we're doing this to make a movie. You're messing up my scene, man."

The cameraman was cuffed first, and only then did the other thieves drop to the ground. The group was arrested and their video was presented to the court as evidence. Two of the men tried to get off by claiming they weren't guilty, but they were on film throwing bricks through the display window.

I don't know if these idiots honestly thought they'd get away with this or not. They loaded more than $2,000 worth of merchandise into their truck and caused about $1,200 worth of damage to the store. They all received community service in lieu of jail time, along with being ordered to pay restitution. I think this was only done because the men hadn't ruined the merchandise and it could still be sold by the boutique.

--I.M.

Nevada

<u>Oink</u>

It's not every day you get called out for a 'violent pig' attack, but I was dispatched to that call.

A male homeowner called 911 to report that he went out to check the mail, when a pig attacked him. He didn't know where the pig came from, but the animal bit his foot.

The man ran inside and told our 911 dispatcher that the pig had then turned on the man's car. It was allegedly chewing on the vehicle. The man stated he was scared and needed help.

I didn't know what to think as the operator played back the 911 feed to my radio. Surely one animal couldn't be that terrifying.

Wrong!

When I exited my vehicle, the pig stopped chewing on the caller's vehicle and charged at me. The pig was pink in color and weighed approximately 80-85 pounds. I tried to jump out of the way, but it grabbed the leg of my pants and refused to let go. I didn't want to shoot it because it looked more like a pet than livestock, so I drew my asp and lightly tapped the pig on its snout to try to release its hold on my leg.

You know what this thing did?

It bit the asp!

As soon as the animal realized it couldn't bite through metal, it lunged at me again. I tried to grab it from behind, but it kept snapping at me and pulling away.

The homeowner came out with a large pillowcase and threw it over the animal. We both tried to subdue it, but it whipped its head around and bit my hand. I could immediately tell the wound would require sutures.

We backed away from the animal and it rushed to the homeowner's porch, leaving us nowhere to go but to my vehicle. I notified dispatch that I needed animal control, and I requested they bring a tranquilizer dart as a backup method.

Luckily, animal control didn't need a tranq dart. They arrived in a van, with the pig's owner. She was crying and kept apologizing. She said the pig hated men and reacted violently to them. She stated she had to take the pet two towns over for vet care because that was the nearest she could find a female vet to handle the pig. She stated she tried to get the pig into 'therapy' for behavioral training, but she couldn't find a dog trainer willing to work with the pig.

We fined the owner for having an animal at large. The pig was quarantined, following the guidelines for a biting dog, and was later released, pending an inspection of his home to prove that the homeowner could contain him to prevent another incident. The homeowner's insurance apparently covered the original caller's vehicle damage and his bite did not require medical attention.

I always thought of pigs as cute and cuddly creatures, but now I know they can be mean when they want to.

--A.R.

Maine

It (Can't) Wait

I had recently begun my shift and needed coffee to survive after a long night of my newborn twins keeping my wife and me awake.

My favorite coffee shop is on a busy side street, so when I parked I didn't think much of the foot traffic, and I didn't pay much attention to these people. One guy stood out as 'maybe I should watch him for a minute,' but I thought I could do that from their patio set *after* I had purchased enough coffee to wake the dead. Besides, the guy wasn't doing anything illegal at the time, just walking. It was his appearance that made me feel uneasy: silver-dollar eyes, messed up hair, not the cleanest skin. I know others think it's bad to 'profile,' but I have to do it if I want to make it home to my family at night. There are times I'm wrong, but when you get that gut feeling, you just should pay attention to that. (For the record, I don't profile based on gender or race; I only try to scan my surroundings for people who seem out of place.)

I ordered my coffee and figured I might as well go to the bakery in the back to pick up a muffin or something while I was there. We don't exactly get scheduled lunch breaks while we're working, and there are more days than others that you don't eat lunch. I hadn't eaten breakfast at home and didn't want to risk having to gnaw my arm off to tide me over until supper.

Someone came inside and I heard the woman ask the barista, "Hey, is that cop in here? I saw a car parked outside."

"I think he's in the back," the barista replied. "Tell him his order's up while you're at it."

I took my 'Double-Trouble Chocolate Muffin with Chocolate Chips' muffin (if I'm going to pay $6.00 for a muffin, I'm not ordering a tasteless bran, okay?) from the pastry clerk and turned to greet the woman who'd been asking about me at the front.

"I'm that cop," I said. "Need something?"

She pointed toward through a row of shelves to the window, "You really need to get out there and do something. It's crazy."

I glanced at my muffin and wondered if I could get away with taking a few bites before I finally decided against it and asked, "What's crazy?"

"Someone's naked in the middle of the road. He peed on a woman walking her dog, and now traffic's stopped."

I placed my muffin on the pastry counter and sighed. It was too early for this crap.

"Oh," the woman said to me, as we walked toward the front, "the cashier said your coffee's ready."

The barista and every customer in the place was face-to-glass when I got to the front of the shop. That's not a good thing for me because that means something serious enough to draw everyone's attention is going down and I have to get involved.

Outside, crowds had gathered on sidewalks. Indeed, there was a nude male in the middle of the road. It was the same guy who gave me an uneasy feeling before I entered the shop. Not only was he nude and blocking traffic as he behaved erratically by alternating between pacing and dancing, but he was shouting and something was on fire behind him.

Grrrrreeeeeat.

"Sir, let's move it off the street and have a talk," I suggested to the man, as I approached him in the middle of one of his 'even a drunk dude at a wedding wouldn't dance that crazy' moves.

He argued and said that if he moved, civilization would end.

"I'd like you to come out of the road peacefully," I stated, growing aggravated. "I don't want to have to use force in this situation."

That was the wrong thing to say, I guess, because this guy started accusing me of working for the Illuminati and said that 'my group' was going to burn down the Pentagon and all kinds of wacky stuff. At one point, this man went from talking about the government and Armageddon to a spiel about how Michael Jackson and Tupac were still alive, being held by the New World Order in Roswell to splice their genes and created a human-alien hybrid race.

I gave the man one last opportunity to move it off the street, but he refused and I moved to arrest him.

This man pulled out moves I didn't even know he had and he roundhouse kicked me in the chest. I fell into the fire that was burning behind us, and it was at this point that I could tell he had burned his clothes in the middle of the road. I was on fire, but I patted myself out and attempted an arrest (again).

It took about five more minutes to arrest this guy and another fifteen to get him in the back of my car. I drove him to the ER and he tested positive for meth.

After medical clearance and sobering up in a cell, he became remorseful of what he could remember, and as I filled him in on what he couldn't recall, he seemed embarrassed. He said he once had a nice apartment, beautiful girlfriend, and great job instructing Jujitsu, but he had fallen on hard times and turned to drugs to get by. I won't ever judge someone for that. It can happen to the best of us. He genuinely seemed interested in turning his life around, and that is the only good thing I can say about this arrest.

I never did get my coffee or my muffin, but thankfully the shop gave me a credit to use for my next visit.

-X.W.

Illinois

Uh...

I routinely patrol a busy tourist location in a city in New York. Most of the time, because of the police presence, crimes are limited in the area. We act as a deterrent, but when we do make arrests or respond to complaints, we are usually stopping a local from harassing a tourist, stopping a drunk tourist from causing unrest in the area, or taking a complaint about a pickpocket or purse theft.

There are days my job is boring. Of course, I walk the area. Sometimes, the other officers and I will get together and have a coffee across the street, but we limit that because we want everyone to know we're more interested in protecting the public than socializing. Most of the time, I stand at one of the local food carts or businesses and get to know the employees, while I people-watch. I've been known to interact with tourists at times, and that can be fun, too.

One day, I was standing by a hot dog cart. Nothing exciting there, right? It was lunchtime and everyone and their brother had to have one of New York's famous dogs (and you should, too, if you ever head our way). I must have watched 100 people come and go for about an hour from this cart. Most people took their food and ate while they walked. Nothing seemed out of the ordinary. I didn't have a reason to suspect anyone for anything. It was a peaceful day with few complaints so far.

I started to see a few women walk by with disgusted looks. Then, I heard a guy yell, "Yo, what the hell is wrong with you, man?"

I tried to stretch my neck to see through the crowd of pedestrians on the sidewalk, but there were too many people.

As I was walking that direction, a woman approached me and said, "Hey, there's a guy doing something gross down there."

I nodded and continued.

In front of thousands of people, a well-dressed man was standing with his back against a diner's window. His pants were unzipped. You're not going to believe what he was doing.

I had seen him, just minutes before, buying a hot dog from the cart I was at. Now, the dog was on the ground, surrounded by splatters of relish and onions. But the bun wasn't.

This man was using the warm bun as a masturbatory tool. His penis was slathered in condiments as he made eye contact with passersby and, for lack of better words, jerked himself off with the bun.

I had a choice here. I could have him turn around and show his penis to the diners inside the café, or I could continue the arrest with the public he'd already to which he'd already exposed himself. Telling him to 'drop the bun and zip up' did nothing. He refused to stop.

The long-story-short here is that I grabbed the wrist of the hand he was using to hold the bun and cuffed him. He didn't resist. I gave him the opportunity to use his other hand to zip up, but he refused again, so I moved him off the sidewalk and stood in front of him until I could get a patrol for transport.

A lot of your stories, I've noticed, end with alcohol or drugs being listed as a factor, but I'm here to tell you that sometimes we just deal with mentally-deranged people. This guy was one of them. It makes what we see just a little more disturbing because I think it's human nature to try to pinpoint a cause for this type of behavior. We *need* to be able to think, 'Oh, nobody would do that. He was drunk? Oh, okay, that makes sense.' The reality of it all is there are people out there who do things like this because they have mental instabilities.

I don't know what happened to the guy after his arrest, and I don't really care to know.

--B.Q.

New York

I once responded to a call from an angry mother who stated her drunk 50-something-year-old neighbor stole her son's tricycle from the front yard and was riding it up and down the sidewalk. He refused to give it back.

He was arrested for public intoxication, theft, and assault, and resisting arrest.

--T.M.

Rhode Island

__Idiot__

I'm assigned as the guard at our courthouse, where all visitors and staff must pass through a metal detector upon entering the building.

One young woman passed through the detector and sounded the alarm.

"Step right over here and please remove anything metal you may be carrying," I stated.

She looked confused and said, "The only thing I have in my pockets is a bag of weed. Should I put that in the basket?"

I smiled and said, "Yes. Yes, you should."

Instant arrest.

Her nipple rings were sounding the alarm. I would have never known about the bag of pot if she hadn't ratted herself out.

-D.N.

Vermont

I once pulled over a driver for operating erratically. As I was approaching the vehicle, he opened the car door and fell out onto the road. What made this worse was that he did not place the vehicle in park, so before it rolled down the ditch, it ran over one of his legs.

Obviously, he was arrested for driving while intoxicated.

--G.K.

Oregon

Be the Change

We all fall on hard times, and I think when you've experienced hitting rock bottom, you're more likely to assist others in crawling out of that deep, dark hole that feels permanent.

I was dispatched to a popular drug store for a report of retail theft. When I arrived, I went to the manager's office and met an adult man who was crying. What he was accused of stealing was placed on the manager's desk. I looked over six 'travel' boxes of tampons, two packages of elastic hair ties, several bottles of trial/travel-size shampoo, and deodorant.

The store manager wanted to press charges.

"You don't strike me as the kind of person who could use tampons," I said to the accused.

He shook his head. "They're for my daughter. She started her period and I couldn't afford to buy them. I didn't know what else to do."

"And what about this other stuff?"

He sobbed and explained that he was having a 'rough year.' His wife had recently passed away and he was left as a single parent to one daughter. He was laid off, which took his financial situation from bad to worse. The bank was in the process of evicting him and his daughter from their home. His truck had broken down. The father had applied for food stamps but was told he made $2.00 more each month than the program would allow to qualify for benefits. Now that he was laid off, he applied for benefits again but was told it could be 'months' for his application to go through. He and his daughter had been getting by, by visiting food pantries. He had contacted a church program for hygienic needs, but the church stated they did not have the items he needed. If he needed diapers or formula, they could have assisted him.

I did what most people don't these days: I sat with this man and *listened*. He apologized a million times for this crime and stated he never thought he would ever resort to breaking the law, but he was trying not to let his bad luck affect his daughter's life. He was having a hard-enough time helping her adjust to living without her mother, and he simply felt he had no alternative in the matter.

I stepped outside the office and spoke to the manager. He was stubborn, but we eventually came to the agreement that he would back down on pressing charges if someone paid for the items and the man would stay away from the business until the time he could come in as a paying customer.

I reentered the office and said to the father, "Okay, let's go."

He didn't care about himself. He cried and said, "Oh, please don't do this. My daughter can't lose both of her parents because I did something stupid."

"Let's go," I said to the man.

He complied and told me, "I'll do anything you need me to do. I know what I did was wrong."

About halfway through the store, I stopped and instructed the man, "Go get a cart and load up on anything you need."

He appeared to be confused.

I motioned to the cart corral. "Go on," I repeated. "Anything you need. Stock up for a while. Maybe get some chips for your daughter to snack on. Get her a pair of fuzzy socks or something. My girls always loved those."

"You don't have to do this," he said.

"I know I don't," I told him. I then explained to him that, before I joined the department, my pregnant wife, my 2-year-old, and I were forced to surrender our dog and cat to a humane shelter, and we were homeless for a month before we were accepted into a shelter. My wife and I had both been laid off from a factory and our only vehicle had broken down. We were drowning in debt after purchasing a money pit and losing a lawsuit with the real estate company. We still had hospital bills from when our first child, my only son, passed away unexpectedly as an infant. By the grace of God, I saw a position listed by the department and applied. For six weeks, my wife and child lived in a shelter, while I was off at training. Some of my pay went towards filing for bankruptcy. The rest went towards getting us into the cheapest, nastiest apartment we could find until we could get back on our feet. It took years, but we succeeded. It may have been decades ago, but I never forgot the feeling of being so down and not being able to provide for my family.

I followed this man around the store and it took ten minutes of nitpicking him for him to open up. He didn't want to put anything in his cart at first, and if he did, he'd choose the cheapest, smallest package of soap or place something in the cart and then place it back on the shelf, saying, "That's not something we really *need*."

An hour later, we went to the register and unloaded toilet paper, snacks, canned food, juice, toiletries, school supplies, and a few 'fun' items. The total was shocking, and it would take a chunk out of my wife's and my savings to go on the cruise we wanted to take, but this needed to be done. I sent the man to wait outside while I purchased him a few gift cards to pizza joints, fast food places, and the store itself.

This man couldn't thank me enough as I left his home after helping him unload all the items we purchased at the store. When

I told the guys at the station about what had occurred, they started a donation pool and our operator called her husband, who is a mechanic. We couldn't do anything about the bank's foreclosure process, but we did help the man fix his vehicle (and it wasn't even as bad as he thought it was), made sure the family was stocked up on groceries, some families donated hand-me-down clothes from their own daughters, and one of our female officers, who the child took a liking to, gave her phone number to the little girl to call if she ever had 'girl problems.'

I checked in with the father occasionally to make sure he was doing okay. The bank took his home, but the man did get hired at a local place and was renting a home owned by his new employer. They may not have had the most luxurious lifestyle, but the two had their basic needs covered, and the father and daughter strengthened their relationship.

Not everyone can do this for someone in need. That's not the point of telling you this story. The point is, the first step is listening and trying to put yourself in that person's position. Just because someone can't provide, doesn't mean that person doesn't want to provide. You could live in a mansion today and be out on the street tomorrow.

You don't have to buy someone groceries or pay their bills or even bring them into your home to help them. Buy them a hot coffee. Sit down and talk to them. Offer a few encouraging words. Not everyone in a bad spot is a bad person or there because they've done something wrong.

All it takes is one person to make a difference. You could be that person.

--C.W.

Location withheld at request

Karma

I don't know if it's because I'm a female officer or I have bad luck or what, but I seem to encounter more 'you're not gonna do anything about it' drivers than my male counterparts when I patrol the highways and interstates.

I was patrolling a rural area and was on a four-lane highway with two lanes each divided by a grassy median. So far that day, I had issued two speeding tickets and one warning for a broken tail light. Because I'm employed as a state trooper instead of local, I catch more attitude from drivers and that day was no exception. I only had a few more hours until my shift was over, thankfully.

I was about five miles behind the nearest cluster of vehicles when a man on a 'pocket rocket' cycle zoomed by me.

Radar indicated the cyclist was traveling at 98 MPH in a 65 MPH zone. I flipped on my lights and siren and accelerated to get nearer to him. This little bastard looked back, flipped me off, and proceeded to speed up. Even then, knowing about the traffic ahead, I didn't know if I'd catch him. His speeds climbed to 120.

As motorists ahead were slow to pull to the side of the road or flat-out failed to do so, the cyclist recklessly weaved in and out of traffic, cutting off other drivers and creating even more of a dangerous environment than he was by speeding alone.

I called out to see if we had anyone patrolling up ahead, but of course we didn't. There was no way in hell I was going to catch this guy. He knew it and I knew it.

I backed off and tried not to let it ruin my already-bad day.

Wouldn't you know it, about five more miles up the road, I rolled up on an accident that other motorists were simply driving around. Skid marks showed the cycle had wobbled before coming to rest on its side near the ditch. The cyclist that had flipped me off a few miles back was now lying on the ground with his helmet split down the middle and his knees busted up and bleeding.

I pulled over and placed my traffic cones before approaching the young man.

"It looks like you took a nasty fall there," I commented.

He was still displaying a nasty attitude and called me a string of expletive-filled names.

I am a nice person. I pride myself on that. If it hadn't been for how he reacted to me when I rolled up on his accident, I think I may have been inclined to call in his MVA as a simple accident and 'forget' that he had evaded me, which is a felony offense. A little niceness goes a long way, doesn't it?

It turned out this kid was only 18 and already had a suspended license, was uninsured, and the bike had been reported as stolen the day before. He also required a medical transport, so he was going to be swimming in legal troubles and debt for a while.

--A.T.

Indiana

What an Idiot!

I was taking a phone report of a stolen bicycle when a man approached my work area, interrupted me, asked, "Hey, is there a place I can smoke?"

Mindlessly, I replied, "Outside, as long as you're twenty-feet away from the entrance. There's a place out there, you'll see it."

I finished the report and was going to pick up our lunch order, so I walked outside and smelled something…illegal.

This is not a joke. This man was standing in the lot's designated smoking area, taking hits from a glass crack pipe.

As I was arresting him, he yelled, "I'm sorry, lady, I thought this was America!"

He tried to fight the drug charges by stating I told him he could smoke. The judge told the subject that he was a moron and threw the book at him.

--L.T.

California

Packing

While I was finishing a theft report at a busy grocery store, a clerk approached me and stated she suspected a teenager of shoplifting. She said she had been stocking and saw the teenager stop repeatedly, open his backpack, and then do this all again a few feet away. I agreed to confront the teenager.

"How are you doing today?" I asked the teenager.

He honestly *did* strike me as the type who would shoplift. I know it's wrong to stereotype, but his hair was dyed some strange color, he had a tattoo that looked real, had multiple facial piercings, wore baggy jeans, and his sure had a vulgar phrase printed on the front. I'm not saying everyone who looks like that would commit a crime, but I wouldn't be surprised to see this kid brought into my precinct.

"Uh, fine," he said.

"Doing a little shopping?"

"Just looking," he replied, refusing to make eye contact.

I laid it out for him. "Look, some of the employees said they saw you open your backpack. They think you may be stealing."

He raised his voice and said, "I'm not. They're liars if they say I am."

"Do you mind if I take a look in your bag?" I asked.

"I don't want you to."

I shrugged, "I'll make you a deal. If you let me look and you're not stealing, but you're carrying something illegal, I'll pretend I didn't see it. As long as it's not a weapon."

"I don't have any weapons. I just don't want to get in trouble."

"Trouble for what?" I asked.

He groaned. "I'm not stealing."

"Then why do you keep opening your backpack? You know, that can look pretty suspicious."

"I have something in there, okay?"

"Like what?" I asked. He wasn't making me think that he was innocent. I hoped he'd just confess to shoplifting and we could let it go before I had to arrest him. I never liked arresting young kids.

"If I show you, will you promise not to arrest me?"

"I already told you," I assured, "as long as you're not stealing and as long as you don't have a weapon, I didn't see anything. I just want to be able to go back up front and tell these employees that you're not stealing merchandise."

"I'm not stealing, I swear."

He carefully removed his backpack and unzipped it.

"Here," he said, motioning me over, "look. I'm not stealing."

I moved in closer and peered into the teenager's pack.

"What the?" I asked. "Why are you carrying that around? Is it wearing a sweater?"

"His name is Percy. He has anxiety, so I knit him sweaters. We go on walks when he's restless, but it started raining and he doesn't like to get wet."

"So, you put a chicken in a backpack and decided to go shopping?"

The teenager nodded. "Yeah, well, until it stops raining. I'll leave, I swear. I'm not stealing. I just can't take him out because I know they'll try to kick us out."

The kid pulled a little rope leash from his pocket and said, "I have this for him, but I don't think they'll let me walk him in here."

I laughed. "Probably not."

"Please don't tell them," the kid begged. "It's a long walk back to my house and I don't want them to kick me out. I have to wait until the rain stops."

I offered to give the kid and his pet chicken a ride back to his house, where the teenager's mom was about to leave for work. She freaked out and thought he was in trouble, until he explained the situation.

That was the weirdest thing I've ever seen.

--A.M.

Arizona

__That Would Explain It__

I pulled a female driver over for speeding and driving erratically.

She argued with me and tried to tell me there wasn't a sign with the posted speed limit.

"Actually," I corrected her, "there is. There *was,* anyway, until you hit it."

"I didn't hit anything," she spat.

"Want to walk back to it?" I offered. "It's just about twenty feet away."

The woman got out of the car and only had on one shoe. She was wearing a shirt that had covered her crotch while she was seated, but when she exited the car, she was nude from the waist down.

"Have you been drinking tonight?" I asked.

She shook her head. "I don't drink."

"Well, is there any reason you don't have pants on, or why you're only wearing one shoe?"

She laughed so hard that she snorted and then *peed* as she was standing up. "I took bath salts."

Well, driving while impaired it was.

--U.D.

West Virginia

<u>We'll Be Right There</u>

This story comes from J.W., with the location withheld at her request. She stated that this 911 call is exactly as she remembers it, and she said she's never laughed so hard in her life.

Operator: 911, please state your emergency.

Caller: Yeah, I think I'm gonna need an ambulance. Probably a firetruck, too.

Operator: Can you tell me what happened?

Caller: Nothing yet.

183

Operator: Sir, are you feeling that you may hurt yourself or another person?

Caller: Yeah, I think I'm going to.

Operator: Sir, are you alone right now?

Caller: Yeah.

Operator: Sir, can you talk to me? Can you maybe talk to me about why you want to hurt yourself? I don't want you to do anything that might hurt yourself. You sound like a very nice man.

Caller: Well, I don't want to hurt myself. That's why I'm calling you. But I don't know what I'm doing, so I'm probably gonna hurt myself.

Operator: We don't want that to happen. What do you mean by you don't know what you're doing?

Caller: Well, I've never made this stuff before. I watched this video on my phone, but it said that if you mess up even one drop, you're probably gonna blow up. And, so, I figured I'd call you guys to send some help. You know, just in case I screw up. Because I probably will screw up.

Operator: Sir, what are you doing? What are you trying to make?

Caller: Crystal meth.

Operator: Sir?

Caller: What?

Operator: You're making crystal meth?

Caller: Trying to.

Operator: And you called 911?

Caller: Yeah.

Operator: Because you're making what?

Caller: Crystal meth.

Operator: Sir, I have a set of gentlemen who are skilled in handling crystal meth. Would you like me to send them to help you?

Caller: You think they could come out? Because I have no idea what I'm doing and don't want to blow myself up.

Operator: Sir, let me get your location and I can guarantee they'll get to you faster than you could ever imagine.

Charges: Too many to even list.

Didn't Think This Through

We received a call regarding a break-in at a local wildlife sanctuary. The office's silent alarm had been tripped and the nearest employee was an hour away, shopping over a long weekend. We were asked if we could secure the area and possibly wait for the employee to arrive. A security guard was on duty, but he was responsible for monitoring security monitors from the multiple guard stations where guards usually allowed or denied vehicular entry. The owner wanted someone with animal experience and office knowledge to be present. We agreed to check it out and wait for someone. The animals there are dangerous, and we didn't want some nutcase or activist to attempt to release the animals.

When we arrived, two windows had been busted out and it was clear someone had attempted to gain entry to a wall safe in the manager's office.

My Sergeant shouted from outside, and I rushed outside to assist. We witnessed a man dressed in all black bolting from the office, running toward a fence to the south.

My Sergeant and I chased after the suspect, calling out for him to stop. He didn't listen, and he was too far ahead for us to deploy a taser. We did not want to fire our weapons.

Against our warnings, the man scaled the high wire fence and dropped down to the open field. He ran to the tree line, as we approached the fence and continued shouting for him to return, hoping he realized his mistake before it was too late.

This facility is a wild cat sanctuary, where tigers, lions, lynx, and other large predators are refuged after surrendered by owners unable to care for them, or after the cats are rescued from abusive situations. Most of the cats are kept in caged habitats and are exercised in a separate field/wooded area on a monitored basis. However, some of the animals are allowed to roam in another field/wooded area, unmonitored. There are signs listed all over the property and it's nearly impossible for anyone to even get on the property. None of the guardrails had been damaged at security checkpoints, and the security guard did not note a vehicle on any of his monitors, so we figured our guy had parked a distance away and had trespassed on foot.

While my Sergeant was calling for assistance and notifying the sanctuary's owners of this issue, I saw our suspect running back to our direction. He was screaming loudly and begging, "Help me. Help me. It's a fucking tiger!"

A tiger emerged from the tree line and just watched the suspect run. The suspect scaled the fence and willingly surrendered for arrest.

The sanctuary owners had a good idea of which tiger the suspect encountered and stated the tiger was generally disinterested in humans and the suspect was lucky that he encountered that tiger, rather than some of the others free-roaming.

--Initials and location withheld at request

I once locked myself out of the house and tried to crawl through the bathroom window.

I got stuck.

Someone driving by thought I was trying to break in, so they called 911 and about half my department showed up because they knew it was my house.

Not only was it embarrassing, but it was also expensive; we had to call someone to cut part of the wall out so they could cut the frame and free me. When they cut, I wriggled free, fell about three feet, and broke my ankle. I had to take seven weeks off work.

--G.G.

Iowa

Do What You Must

I arrived at a residence after a frantic 911 call from an elderly woman. She stated someone had broken into her home, and her husband had killed the intruder. Our operator was having a difficult time keeping the caller calm, and at one point the woman stated she was having chest pains, so EMS was also dispatched.

When I entered the home, I saw a man in his twenties sprawled out on the hallway floor. He was bleeding from his head.

I was going to check that man for a pulse, but the elderly male homeowner was lying on the floor, sobbing, and clutching his chest. His wife was kneeled at his side, and she was also crying. She told me she was sure she and her husband were both having heart attacks. She had taken a nitro pill and gave her husband one. A very large, very fluffy dog sat between the two and took turns licking its owners.

I attempted to calm the couple, but the two kept talking between each other. It took a minute or two, but finally I could tell between their cries that they were promising to love each other, even when the husband went to prison for the rest of his life. They honestly believed I would arrest the husband for murder and that he would spend his remaining days in prison, and the wife said that it would all be okay because she would go live with one of their children (I assumed that's who they were talking about, anyway).

"I need you folks to tell me exactly what happened," I stated.

"I should probably get a lawyer first," said the man.

"Just tell him. Our lives are over, anyway," his wife wept.

"I hit him with Milo's bone."

"A bone?" I asked. I looked around. "Where is it?"

"Milo is very protective of his bone. After I dropped it, Milo grabbed it. It's probably in his bed or behind my recliner. He likes to squeeze back there and hide it."

Milo licked my face.

"But, a bone?"

"It was the only thing I could think to use to defend myself," the man answered. "Oh, please. If you're going to arrest me, please don't do it in front of my wife."

EMS arrived and I moved to check vitals on the bleeding intruder.

He wasn't dead; he was knocked out cold.

While EMS was loading everyone up, I walked through the house with the intention of bagging the bone for evidence. I was incredibly surprised to find (behind the recliner, just like his owner stated) a

19-inch-long smoked beef bone that weighed about six pounds. That gash on the intruder's head sure made a lot more sense than when I was imagining the elderly man smacking the intruder with a tiny rawhide.

EMS transported everyone to the hospital, and it was there that a nurse recognized the intruder as someone who was wanted in another county for a string of burglaries. She had seen a post on Facebook.

Luckily, this all worked out. The intruder was given six sutures and was hauled to jail.

We didn't charge the homeowners with a crime because they were well within their rights of protecting their home, especially after the full version of the home invasion came to light and we heard the intruder pulled a knife on the couple.

Unfortunately, both homeowners suffered from heart attacks and the wife underwent surgery. I visited her husband on the CCU wing and he apologized for what he did, but he did what he had to do to keep his family safe.

--J.O.

Montana

I Work Out

Dispatch notified me that a caller reported that she witnessed a male parked in his car at a closed church camp, and the male was allegedly masturbating. She admitted she had not seen the male's penis, but she lived across the road from the rural camp and was watching the teenager with a pair of binoculars. She said there was no way he was doing anything else and 'he's been doing it for a few minutes.'

Well, that's no Bueno.

It took virtually no time for me to get there, so at midnight, I pulled into the church camp drive and immediately saw a parked vehicle. A startled male teen driver locked a terrified stare with me as I parked, fully knowing he couldn't go anyplace. I saw him look down and scramble to do something with his hands. I figured he was zipping up.

I approached the vehicle and knocked on the window. The teenager inside couldn't have been older than 16 or 17. He was a scrawny little guy.

"I'm sorry," he blurted out. "I'm sorry."

"You're sorry? You think that's enough for touching yourself in public? You do know someone saw you, right?"

The kid looked confused. "Huh? Touching myself?"

He spoke frantically. "Oh, God. Oh, can I say that here? I probably shouldn't say that here. Oh, God, I'm going to go to Hell."

"Let's try to breathe," I said.

"I wasn't touching myself, though."

"If you're not touching yourself, can you explain why you're out here trespassing in the middle of the night?"

The teenager's eyes went glossy and filled up with tears. "I don't want to tell you."

"If you don't tell me, I'm going to take you in for trespassing. We'll call your parents, and then they'll have to hear about it, too. Look, I'm not in the mood for games tonight, so how about you just tell me what you were doing, and let me decide how I'm going to handle it, okay?"

The teen's lower lip quivered, and he said, "It's under my seat."

I stepped back and asked him to exit the vehicle. He obeyed orders as I instructed him to stand in front of his car, though by this time he was sobbing.

I put on a glove and cautiously reached under the driver's seat until I felt something large and circular. I pulled it out and shined my flashlight on it. I was holding the end of a Shake Weight.

I held it up and asked the boy, "This? This is what you were doing?"

"Jane Doe says I have Frosty the Snowman arms!" he shouted through his loud cries. Snot shot out his nostrils.

I must be a horrible person because I don't think I've ever laughed harder in my life. I couldn't see because I had tears, and I could hardly breathe. My stomach cramped up and I had to sit down sideways in the kid's driver's seat to catch my breath. All the while, I guess he had stopped crying and just kind of looked at me like I was the biggest jerk in the world.

After I caught my breath, I asked the kid why in the world he'd come out to an empty church camp to do that, and he said, "Because if I did it anywhere else everyone would laugh at me like you did."

Man, I felt like a horrible person, but I just couldn't stop chuckling.

Before I told the boy to go home, I told him it's common for teen boys to develop muscle definition at different times, and that he still had time to work out properly and see definition over time. He asked for a few workout tips and said he wanted to join a gym but didn't want to be teased, so I told him he couldn't avoid that because you can't control how others act, you can only control how you react.

Since nothing ever happens around here, that's been my favorite response of my time in this area. I feel bad for making the kid feel insecure, but I still laugh when I think about the kid just sitting in the dark using a Shake Weight hard enough for someone to make a 911 call.

--D.X.

Ohio

<u>Back in Time</u>

I was patrolling when I witnessed a man in his 30s attempting to gain access to a newspaper machine on a street corner.

"What are you doing?" I asked, as I pulled up beside him.

"Trying to find out what year it is," he screamed, drawing attention of pedestrian traffic on the sidewalks.

Okay, that's a pretty good indication that I need to actually get out of the car to talk to the guy.

I moved around to speak with the guy, and he was freaking out. He kept looking around like he couldn't believe his surroundings, and he kept making comments about my radio and cell phones people were talking on as they passed. For example, he would chuckle and say,

"Yeah, I remember when those were popular."

My first question was, "Have you been drinking?"

He said no.

"Have you used any form of drug?"

Again, no.

I asked the man if he had an ID on him, to which he stated he didn't. I then asked him if he had a place to go for the night, and he said, "I don't know. I don't know if my house has been built yet."

I suggested that we visit the hospital to have someone 'check him out,' which was my code for 'you really need a psych eval,' but he refused and then started yelling at pedestrians, asking what year it was and if they had random electronics that really just sounded like he took two or three different modern-day brand names and mashed them together to create a 'future' brand. I couldn't tell if he was high as a kite or just had a few screws loose upstairs.

I told the man I was arresting him for disturbing the peace and felt he needed medical attention. When he went to the hospital, they seemed to agree. The man was tested for drugs, but nothing was found in his system, so he was placed on the mental health wing for overnight observation.

Someone checked in with me the next day and told me the man wasn't mentally ill; he had consumed magic mushrooms, which don't leave traces on the tests the hospital administers. The man had no idea how he ended up in the hospital and thought he had overdosed. He said it was his first time trying the shrooms, and I guess it was also his last. We agreed to drop charges.

That's not the craziest thing I've encountered on the job, but it is probably the safest one I could probably send to you.

--I.P.

Nevada

I've lost count on how many people yell, "Just arrest me, then!" and then act surprised when I actually arrest them.

What did you think I was going to do?

--T.R.

Kentucky

Brave

Neighbors called to report theft in progress at a home. The homeowners were at work, and two to three men were reported leaving the home with the owners' possessions.

When I arrived, the yard was a mess. There was a pickup parked on the lawn, with televisions and furniture loaded in the bed. To my right was a washer and behind that was a dryer. There were clothes and things that wouldn't be considered valuable to a criminal lying on the ground. Two old Yorkies were following a man as he exited the house with a box in his arms. He froze when he saw me.

"I think we both know you're busted," I said to the man. "Why don't you surrender peacefully?"

"Busted for what?" he snarled. "You can't arrest me."

I laughed. "I know this isn't your house. You and your buddies are something else, trying to pull this off in broad daylight on a weekday."

Another man emerged from the home, carrying a small fish tank.

"Oh crap," he moaned. "Someone called the cops?"

"Yeah," the other guy said. "But I was just telling him that he couldn't arrest us because we're having a yard sale."

I looked around. "You're having a yard sale?"

"Yeah," said the first man. "Anything you want, just shoot me a price and it's yours."

Unbelievable.

This exchange went on for a few more minutes, until I asked the guys what their dogs were named. They answered simultaneously, giving two sets of names each.

I was surprised neither tried to run before I placed them under arrest. One of the neighbors had called the homeowners, and the female arrived just as I was calling someone to come watch the residence and get a tow truck to remove the thieves' pickup from the lawn.

Most of the homeowners' belongings were salvageable, except for a few clothes that were stained by mud and grass. The woman thanked me and moved her dogs inside, all the while scolding them.

"Do you want to show them where we keep the nice silverware, too?" I heard her ask them.

--K.N.

South Carolina

Tell It How It Is

I understand some individuals fear or distrust law enforcement. Some believe we, as officers, want to take away the publics' rights to live freely. Others believe we, as a collective, possess no respect for life and will pull the trigger as soon as we have the chance, just because we have the chance. We hear constantly that we're 'only pulling you over to meet a quota' for citations issued. We hear 'fuck the police' as we patrol through neighborhoods.

Some of us do not make it home. A father of three may leave his house in the morning, after kissing his pregnant wife goodbye, unknowing to the fact that he will be shot twice in the chest during a routine traffic stop, during which he had already decided before even pulling the vehicle over that he was only going to issue a warning because 'he was having a good day.' Wives and mothers leave their children in their beds at night and are beaten to death while responding to a trivial complaint, like a resident locked out of his apartment.

As in any field, there are some bad officers out there: bad at upholding the law, bad at possessing compassion, bad at making rushed decisions, bad at maintaining integrity, or bad at understanding that we are all human beings striving to survive. Unfortunately, those officers disgrace our entire profession and give us all a bad name.

That is not who I am. That is not who my coworkers and brothers and sisters in arms are. That is not who most officers are.

I took this job because my father was murdered for the two-dollars he had in his wallet. I was five-years-old when the mugger shot my father in the stomach and then put the loaded gun against my forehead. I wanted help. I needed help. But nobody came. From then on, I knew I wanted to prevent that kind of situation from happening to another child, another wife, husband, nephew, grandparent. I wanted to rid the streets of criminals so that others could live in peace, so my mother could walk to the grocery store without feeling that the man walking behind her would kill her and leave her body on the sidewalk.

Our dispatcher took her job because she lived in an apartment complex where dealers tried to sell her six-year-old ecstasy. She now lives in a two-bedroom house in a quiet neighborhood and said that dispatching became a way of coping because she didn't have a way to control life at home. She needed this job as much as it needed her.

The world is filled with bad people, and it hurts me to think that officers are lumped in that group, when most of us are trying to clean up a never-ending mess and just make it home after a long day of being spit on, cussed at, shot at, or lead on foot patrols for a mile and a half.

I can't speak for the bad officers, and I won't because I find them just as detestable as the rest of the nation does. Please, though, believe me when I say that the rest of us, the majority, are with the department to keep you safe, to help you escape from a bad situation, to help you live in peace.

--C.E.

New Jersey

Awww

If stories went 'viral' thirty years ago like they do today, I would be famous for what happened to me.

We routinely visited a residence for complaints of drugs, domestic disputes, animal and dependent neglect, and noise complaints. The domestic disputes worsened after dependents were removed from the home, but I think we all saw that one coming. The calls didn't slow down. It didn't seem like there was an end in sight.

One of the neighbors called in yet another complaint of noise at the residence and stated she may have heard someone screaming from inside the home, so I headed out, thinking this would either be an open and shut case of, "Fine, I'll turn the damn music down," or "You're under arrest for domestic battery."

I knocked on the door three times before the husband answered. His clothes were ratty and dirty. The living room was crawling with bugs. In the corner were two pit bull-mixes, painfully underweight and mistreated, but the local humane society said the process of removing animals from the home was tough. The man's wife was naked, lying on the couch with a joint in her hand. I could have arrested her for marijuana possession, but I'm a little more lenient on pot because I smoked so much of it as a teenager.

"I've had complaints about some noise again tonight," I said.

"Because she's watching that goddamn TV as loud as it'll go," the man grunted.

"Because you won't shut the hell up and let me watch," the wife retorted.

216

"Can we try to maybe keep it down?" I asked.

The husband picked up what appeared to be days-old chicken from a KFC bucket and began chomping on a breast. As he was flipping the piece over, he dropped it to the ground and the dogs bolted from the corner to snatch it up from the dirty floor.

Without missing a beat, the man reached down and punched one of the dogs in the temple and kicked the other one in the stomach.

"I'm going to go ahead and place you under arrest for animal abuse," I told him.

This made him scream out a long line of expletives and threats to me, and he finally said, "Just tell someone to take them. I don't even want the damn things."

I could have continued with my plan to place the man under arrest, but I decided to do one better. I told him I would leave with the dogs.

"Take 'em," he shrugged. "I don't give a shit. They're mean, anyway, and they don't listen for a damn."

"I'd imagine the way you treat them has something to do with that," I responded.

The man went off on me again, telling me it was none of anyone's business how he treated the dogs and dogs are meant to obey at all times.

I asked for the dogs' names, to which the wife laughed from the couch and said, "We just call them dogs."

Neither dog would budge from the corner, so I took off my jacket and wrapped one in it, planning to return for the second after I placed the first in my car. I didn't have to return because the second dog willingly followed as soon as I lifted the first from the ground. I noticed immediately that the dogs were covered in fleas and appeared to have burn marks. Their fur was falling out in patches and when my jacket slipped, I could feel the first dog's bones through its skin.

My first order of business was taking the animals to the vet at nearly midnight. I didn't know what I was going to do with two dogs, but I figured the first step of removing them from the home was as good as it was going to get at that point.

At the vet's office, the dogs were both found to be heartworm negative, but they were infested with worms and it took two flea dips each to kill the parasites. Both dogs showed evidence of long-term abuse, but externally and internally. X-rays showed both dogs, at one point, had sustained fractures to their ribs, hips, and legs. The burns on both dogs were thought to be from cigarettes put out on their skin. I stayed at the vet's office for five hours as the vet and his assistants tried to clean up the dogs. The entire time, the dogs refused to be separated and would howl and yip if they couldn't see one another.

I asked what would happen to them when it was time to leave, and the vet scowled. He said the dogs would be turned over to the humane shelter, but it was unlikely they would be adopted because of their breed, and the fact that they were abused would scare potential adopters away. I knew the likelihood of both dogs being adopted by the same family was slim, if even a family took one. The vet told me if the dogs weren't adopted after a week, they would be euthanized.

I should have called my wife to run it by her, but the plan was so sudden that I wasn't sure what I was doing, even as I pulled in the driveway with two frightened dogs in my backseat.

My wife met me at the front door (I'm surprised she wasn't holding the rolling pin), thinking that I had been so late returning home because I went out to drink and play poker. She was pleasantly surprised to see me carry in one of the dogs and to see the second timidly following. She dropped to the hall floor and both dogs eventually moved to her and allowed her to pet them, though they would often flinch or run away and hide in the corner.

We named the dogs Remington and Steele after my wife's favorite television program at the time.

With time, the dogs learned they were in a safe, loving environment. They went from skin and bones to maybe a bit on the pudgy side, and they quickly became pros at learning how to beg at the table efficiently. My wife made each dog a bed, but they only used one at a time. They refused to do anything separately.

My wife fell pregnant that year and we welcomed my daughter. We were admittedly cautious about having previously-abused animals in a home with an infant, but the dogs took to that baby like sticky to gum, and they never left her side. They went from sleeping in their bed in the television room, to sleeping on her bed when she was old enough to be moved from a crib. Over the years, they allowed her to dress them, loved protecting her as she learned to ride a bike, and they'd swim with her when we went to the lake during summers.

I don't know what happened to the scum that abused the dogs; I don't care. We responded to complaints for years, but then they moved away.

The dogs the couple surrendered lived long, happy lives. We worked on training the duo and proving to them that humans can love another creature. They were the best dogs I've ever had in my life. My only regret involving the dogs is that we couldn't remove them from the home sooner. It still pains me to think that they endured such a tremendous amount of abuse, and it amazes me that they both came out of that type of environment, still capable of loving and protecting.

Both dogs passed away at ripe old ages, and I still miss them terribly.

--O.L.J.

Illinois

Imagine our surprise when a man walked in our station at 03:00 and confessed that he was Jack the Ripper!

He looked good, I mean, for committing murders in late-1800s.

We stuck him in the drunk tank until he sobered up.

--T.P.

Delaware

If I get one more subpoena for a call I didn't even respond to, I might be able to use my comp time to retire 20 years earlier than planned.

--M.O.

Florida

Law Enforcement Oath of Honor

On my honor, I will never betray my badge, my integrity, my character, or the public trust.

I will always have the courage to hold myself and others accountable for our actions.

I will always uphold the constitution, my community, and the agency I serve.

<u>A Message to Readers</u>

I didn't plan to release an LEO version of this series until I noticed how many submissions I received from officers. I tried something new this time around, by limiting the sad/dramatic stories and using as many feel-good submissions as I could find. With everything going on in the world today, that just felt like the right thing to do. As you probably noticed quickly, many of these submissions are not medical in nature, but I felt they should be shared, anyway.

I hope you all have enjoyed this edition. I thought about throwing in a story from the fire department at the end, just to poke fun at the lighthearted rivalry we hear about between officers and firefighters, but I decided against it at the last moment.

In all seriousness, I have nothing but respect for officers and supporting staff on the force. These men and women go above and beyond the call of duty each day, and I support them 100-percent. As one of the submissions mentioned, every profession has its share of bad seeds, and law enforcement is not exempt. Especially with everything going on out there, I can only hope the goodness outweighs the bad and that we can all find peace and understanding during these difficult and confusing times.

I have been sorting through submissions for a condensed Winter reader-submission edition. While I'm not working on that, I've been poking and prodding at some other work, but I'm not confident enough to release some of that, and other stuff I've been working on is taking forever and a day because it involves tons of research and carefully setting the mood and setting for historical accuracy. Who know when (or if) some of those pieces will be finished and/or released. I will never release something to you unless I can stand behind it confidently.

I want to continue to shout out a hearty 'THANK YOU!' to all readers, established and new to the series and my other works. I couldn't have done any of this without you, and I do enjoy interacting with you on social media. I appreciate you all.

For all of you affected by the terrible tragedies taking place right now, I pray for your safety and for your peace of mind. Please do your best to keep yourselves safe and know you are never alone in your battles.

Have a great day, everyone!

Check me out on Twitter!

https://twitter.com/AuthorKerryHamm

My website:

http://www.authorkerryhamm.com

I'm also on Facebook. Drop a search for Author Kerry Hamm to find my page!

Made in the USA
Columbia, SC
02 May 2019